The Wheat-Free Journey

Amazing Dishes for your Wheat-Free Lifestyle

Table of Contents

Introduction

Wheat Free Pancakes with Berry Topping

Sugar Free Baked Apples

Very Berry Fruit Cereal

Chopped Spicy Zucchini

Lunch Cookbook

Squash with Sliced Mushroom

Zucchini Onion Rolls

Avocado & Tomato Pizza

Red & Yellow Pepper Pizza

Easy Spicy Eggplant Dish

Nutty Harvest Boat

Cucumber Raft

Ratatouille Riverboat

Fruitychicken Melonboat

Barreling Down the River

Red Wrap

Spicy Seafruit Wraps

Dragonchicken Wraps

Eggplant Chicken Burgers

Chickenfish Wraps

Mangospice Chicken Soup

Earthroot Soup

Omelet Soup

Trail Mix Soup

Honeyfruit Soup

Dinner Cookbook

Lemon Chicken & Vegetable Blend

Chopped Chicken & Veggie Salad

Delicious Baked Juicy Meat

Spicy Stewed Steaks

Oven Cooked Vegetable & Stew Blend

Mirepoix with Red Sauce

Quick Asian Veggie Soup

Spicy Oregano Cubes

Lamb Slits

Spicy Kale Quiche

Red Pepper Chicken Fries

Nuts & Turkey Burgers

Sugar Free Meat Drizzle

Chickplant Filets

Chicken Bruschetta

Eggplant with Pesto Topping

Salmon with Berry Chutney

Spicy Zucchini Eggplant Dine

Lettuce Nut Salad

Baked Tilapia Filets

Comfort Food Cookbook

Pancake Bacon Breakfast

Breakfast steak and Eggs

Midnight Chicken and Waffles

Avocado Egg Salad

Grilled Cheese Sandwich

Cheesy Southern Jalapeño "Cornbread"

Chili Con Carne

Sweet Potato Cheese Fries

Portobello Overload Burger

Spicy Meatballs and Tomato Sauce

Pan-Fried Eggplant Parm

Cashew Ricotta Lasagna

Italian Sausage and Peppers

Cashew Mac and "Cheese"

Delicious Chicken Pot Pie

Little Lamb Sheppard's Pie

Country Chicken and Dumplings

All Day Country Fried Steak

Bacon Sautéed Liver and Onions

Oven-Crunch Chicken

Garlicky Mashed Parsnips

Oven-Crisp Croquettes

Tropical Beef Patty

Sweet Banana Bread

Pumpkin Spice Bread

Asian Cookbook

Cashew Chicken Satay

Savory BBQ Pork Bun

Easy Kimchi

Japanese Seaweed Salad

Asian Meatball Snacks

Chinese Orange Chicken

Sweet and Sour Chicken Bites

Asian Style Calamari

Triple Cashew Chicken

Zucchini Noodle Pad Thai

Mei Fun

Fresh Noodle Chicken Chow Fun

Thai-Style Coconut Chicken

Sesame Chicken

Classic General Tso's Chicken

Indian Egg Fried Rice

Chicken and Cashew Stir-Fry

Spicy Beef and Broccoli

Tender Grilled Korean Beef

Stir-Fried Mongolian Beef

Asian Orange Roasted Duck

Braised Spare Ribs

Coconut Lime Thai Steamed Mussels

Asian Mustard Baked Salmon

Coconut Egg Custard Tartlets

Sweet Treat Cookbook

Sweet Cinnamon Breakfast Rolls

Lavender and Lemon Scones

Scrumptious Cherry Pie

Southern Strawberry Pie

Mixed Berry Cobbler

Coconut Egg Custard Pie

Apricot Meringue Pie

Southern Peach Cake

Raisin Pecan Cake

Coconut Pineapple Cake

Caramel Banana Cake

Lemon Chiffon Bundt Cake

Freezer Chocolate Cheesecake

Banana Shortbread Cookies

Sweet Tea Biscuits

Tart Almond Cookies

Nut Raisin Cookies

Baked Ginger Pudding

Indian Sweet Laddu

Stove-Top Almond Fudge

Asian Sesame Cookie Crisps

Fruit-Filled Chinese Moon Cakes

Churros and Chocolate Sauce

Coconut Custard Flan

Coconut Jelly

Snacks Cookbook

Spicy Sweet Potato Brittle

Celery with Baby Carrots

Wheat Free Fruit Cookies

Wheat Free Cashew Coconut Balls

Cool Berry Drink

Icy Blueberry Delight

Strawberry Blend

Chunked Apples

Baked Cauliflower

Almond & Banana Bar

Black Pepper & Kale Chips

Chocó Raisins

Creamy Raspberry

Mixed Fruit Drizzle

Fruits Blend

Broccoli Fries

Nuts & Raisin Bars

Orange Nutmeg Treat

Rich Mixed Fruit Creamy Salad

On the Go Cookbook

Strawberry Breakfast Pastry

Orange Anzac Cookies

Cocoa Zucchini Muffin

Crunchy Almond Butter Granola Bar

Raw Island Sweet Bread

Soft Baked Poppy Seed Pretzel

Superfood Granola

Salt and Vinegar Dehydrated Kale Chips

Caribbean Jerked Beef Jerky

Fennel Seed Flax Crackers

Chocolate Nib Trail Mix

Tart Cherry Lime Energy Bar

Blueberry Licorice Fruit Rolls

Traditional Almond Macarons

Sweet Vanilla Shortbread Biscuits

Cherry Fig Newton Cookies

Lemon Coconut Pinwheels

Raisin Cinnamon Rugalach

Cranberry Pistachio Biscotti

Double Chocolate Scone

Sweet Almond Balls

Sesame Seed Date Balls

Salted Pretzel Rods

Honey and Spice Nuts

Pecan Pie Brittle

Meat Cookbook

All-Natural Chicken Sausage

Gourmet Turkey Legs

Classic Rack of Lamb with Mint Sauce

Modern Beef Haggis

Bacon Filet Mignon Steak

Beef Braciole with Tomato Sauce

Roasted Stuffed Game Hen

BLT Burger Wrap

Baked Pork Chops with Cinnamon Apples

Veal Scallopini with White Wine Sauce

Simple enison Stir-Fry

Bison Bacon Burger

Amazing Bacon Dog with Rémoulade

Pork Tenderloin with Apricot Sauce

Gourmet Chicken Liver Pâté

Crispy Pan Seared Duck

Cajun Spice Broiled Gator Tail

Veggie Medley Stuffed Peppers

Walnut Sausage Stuffed Tomatoes

Sautéed Frog Legs with Lemon Butter Sauce

Healthy Gyro

Greek Souvlaki Kebobs

Beef Stuffed Cabbage in Tomato Sauce

Homestyle Sunday Meatloaf

Brazilian Churrasco with Chimichurri

Holiday Cookbook

Sweet and Tart Cranberry Sauce

"Green Bean" Casserole

Tender Collard Greens

Christmas Skillet "Cornbread"

Sage "Cornbread" Dressing

Sweet Candied Yams

Pineapple Spice Baked Ham

Perfect Roasted Turkey

Homestyle Sweet Potato Pie

Holiday Apple Crumble

Delicious Fruit Cake

Sweet Pumpkin Cheesecake

Harvest Spice Cake

Sweet Date Gingerbread Cookies

Warm Spiced Mulled Wine

Coconut Milk Eggnog

Sweet Horchata

Sweet Mango Lassi

Pan Asian Mushroom Masala

Indian Sweet Fig Pudding

Asian Holiday Spiced Nuts

French Holiday Tapenade

Hanukkah Sweet Potato Latkes

Lots o' Matzo Ball Soup

Festival Cherry Nut Rugelach

Why Eat Wheat-Free?

Wheat has been a staple of our diet for generations. Pies, bread, cookies, all fresh from the oven, were featured at meals in our grandmothers' days. This is even truer today with the heavy consumption of sandwiches and wraps, couscous, pasta, pizza, baked goods, snack bars and breaded meat. Leading nutritionists are recommending whole wheat as a healthy source of whole grains, claiming it lowers the risk of heart disease and promotes weight loss. But just how healthy is wheat?

As it turns out, it may not be as healthy as we've made it to be in the last few decades. Like all grains and plant foods, wheat contains both protein and carbohydrates. Its high carbohydrate content provides some quick energy while the protein digests more slowly and helps keep hunger at bay for a few hours. Unfortunately, the protein found in wheat, known as gluten, is now thought to be especially harmful to humans. In about 1% of the population, eating gluten triggers a severe auto-immune reaction that causes their bodies to attack their small intestines and destroy the tiny finger-like projections called villi. The villi's role is to increase the surface area of the small intestine's membrane in order to absorb nutrients from partially digested food. When the villi are destroyed by antibodies, the surface area is greatly reduced and the intestine can no longer absorb nutrients properly. The person becomes sick from malnourishment, despite a normal and healthy diet.

This disease, known as Celiac disease, is the extreme version of gluten intolerance. For most Celiacs, a crumb of bread is enough to destroy their intestines, and the damage takes several weeks or even months to heal.

The only known treatment is a strictly gluten-free diet that eliminates all traces of wheat, rye and barley. Awareness on the subject of wheat and gluten intolerance is quickly spreading. Many believe that as much as 20 to 30% of the population suffers from gluten intolerance or non-Celiac gluten sensitivity (NCGS). These are usually milder versions of Celiac disease without the destruction of villi. However, the gluten sensitivity spectrum is broad and ranges from mildly sensitive (gas, bloating) to nearly-Celiac with the whole array of gluten-related symptoms. Some people also suffer from a wheat allergy, which causes an immediate and life-threatening condition known as anaphylactic shock.

But why are people so sensitive to wheat today when this food has been around for so long? The truth is, it hasn't been around that long at all. It was merely 10,000 years ago that humans discovered agriculture; they started growing crops and raise livestock, which became new staples in their diet. These 10,000 years are hardly significant on the evolution timeline, and experts believe that our bodies did not have time to adapt to this sudden intake of grain-based products. This has worsened in the last half-century, as modern advances in technology have allowed us to create new species of wheat that yield more crops and contain twice as much gluten as before. Gluten makes wheat products sticky and traps air in tiny bubbles, giving baked goods their nice soft and airy texture. Extra gluten creates fluffier and chewier bread, which in turn sells better to consumers. This increased intake of gluten and wheat-based products is making many people sick. In fact, wheat and milk rank as the two top allergens found in today's food!

Gluten breaks down into different smaller proteins which cannot be digested properly and leak through the small intestine, causing inflammation throughout the body. This inflammation has been linked to many modern diseases that are seemingly unrelated, such as cancer, Alzheimer's disease, diabetes, obesity and ADHD. On top of gastrointestinal symptoms such as diarrhea and cramps, gluten intolerance in general is also linked to infertility, migraines, eczema, allergies, fatigue and hundreds of other symptoms. For these reasons, many people could greatly benefit from adopting a wheat-free and gluten-free lifestyle.

There is no single approach that works for everyone when talking about wheat and gluten. Some people who are mildly sensitive could get away with reducing gluten intake, or switching to grains with less gluten in them (rye and barley, along with ancient forms of wheat such as kamut and spelt). Others, such as Celiacs and those suffering from severe NCGS need to avoid all traces of gluten.

If you suspect you have an intolerance to gluten and are interested in trying a wheat-free lifestyle, this book can greatly help you. Giving up wheat can be hard at first, and there is a learning curve involved. But, thousands of people feel much better after eliminating wheat from their diet. While it is a good source of some nutrients, wheat is far from irreplaceable. There are hundreds of naturally wheat-free options that provide the nutrition you need on a daily basis. Of course, it can be tempting to rush to the store and buy out the entire section of gluten-free products. The truth about these products is shocking: on average, they contain more calories, more fat and more sugar than their wheat-based counterparts and provide very little nutrition.

A balanced wheat-free lifestyle restricts the use of prepared gluten-free products to special occasions only. Emphasize meat, veggies, nuts, eggs and seeds, add a little rice or quinoa and some fresh herbs. By eliminating wheat, you will discover a whole new way of cooking that features wholesome and fresh foods instead of processed white flour. This guide contains many recipes to help you transition to a wheat-free lifestyle. If you suspect severe gluten intolerance, make sure you get properly diagnosed as you may need to eliminate all traces of gluten from your diet. Indeed, about 90% of Celiacs are currently undiagnosed and destroy their intestines on a daily basis by ingesting wheat and gluten.

Cooking without wheat is an interesting challenge and leads you to exploring some foods you might not have thought about before. You can recreate nearly anything without wheat. Usually, the results will be different because the lack of gluten changes the texture of food. However, as with any other lifestyle, it will become the new normal. The recipes in this book are Celiac-friendly, meaning they contain absolutely no gluten ingredients. They are also free of processed ingredients such as white sugar, table salt, grain starches and artificial flavors. But, ultra-healthy doesn't have to mean boring; we guarantee you'll love your new lifestyle!

Foods to Avoid

You will want to avoid:

- Wheat bread, whether it's white bread, whole wheat or multigrain. This includes other types of bread such as rolls, hot dog buns, flour tortillas, naan, pita wraps, pretzels and fruit breads.
- Most pasta, pizza crusts and gnocchi, as they are made with wheat flour.
- Anything breaded, such as meat tenders, mozzarella sticks and tempura, as the breading is usually wheat-based.
- Baked goods such as muffins, cake, granola bars, soft snack bars, cookies, wafers, etc. Make your own at home with no wheat; nut flours and coconut flour make amazing and nutritious baked goods.
- Soy sauce: most commercial soy sauce, including the soy sauce used in prepared Asian dishes, is fermented with the use of wheat. Try to find tamari soy sauce, which is darker and richer in flavour than regular soy sauce and contains no wheat.
- Sauces and gravies: they are usually thickened with wheat flour. Find gluten-free gravies or make your own at home.
- Glucose syrup: it is often made from wheat. Gluten is generally removed by all the processing, allowing companies to label it as gluten-free. However, if it's made with wheat, it can still cause reactions in some people. Glucose syrup is very processed and unhealthy and should be avoided anyway.

- Pre-packaged and processed foods: not only are they loaded with sugar and preservatives, these foods often contain wheat-based ingredients.
- Kamut, spelt and triticale: the first two are ancient forms of wheat while triticale is a cross between wheat and rye. In wheat-sensitive people, these grains can trigger the same reactions as regular wheat.
- Fake meats and seitan: vegan meat substitutes usually contain gluten as one of their primary sources of protein. Seitan is pure gluten, and should be avoided at all costs.
- Couscous: most couscous is made from wheat.
- Wheat by-products such as wheat germ and bran
- Oats: this grain is inherently gluten-free, but it's usually harvested and processed in close association with wheat. Even pure, uncontaminated oats will sometimes trigger a gluten sensitivity response in certain people.

Breakfast Cookbook

Celery Blend with Spinach

Green smoothie with a variety of vegetables.

Prep time: 5 minutes

INGREDIENTS

1 handful spinach

½ avocado

1 banana

1 large stalk celery

1 tbsp coconut oil

1 tsp cinnamon

1 cup water

INSTRUCTIONS

1. Slice avocado in half and remove the nut. Break the banana into small pieces and chop the celery into small pieces.

2. Combine all ingredients except for the spinach into a blender. Blend them until pureed, then add spinach and blend until pureed.

3. Serve or chill and then serve.

Fruit Blend in a Natural Cup

Sweet, creamy smoothie with a combination of fruits and vegetables.

Prep time: 5 minutes

INGREDIENTS

1 handful spinach

½ avocado

1 banana

½ cup blueberries

1 tbsp coconut oil

1 tsp cinnamon

1 cup water

INSTRUCTIONS

1. Slice avocado in half and remove the nut. Break the banana into small pieces.
2. Combine all ingredients except for the spinach into a blender. Blend them until pureed, then add spinach and blend until pureed.
3. Serve or chill and then serve.

Garden Vegetable Refresher

Green smoothie with a variety of hearty vegetables.

Prep time: 5 minutes

INGREDIENTS

1 handful Kale

1 banana

1 large cucumber

1 handful green beans

1 tbsp coconut oil

1 tsp cinnamon

1 cup water

INSTRUCTIONS

1. Break the banana into small pieces. De-stem the kale, skin and chop the cucumber and de-stem the green beans.

2. Combine all ingredients except for kale in a blender. Blend them until pureed, then add kale and blend until pureed.

3. Serve or chill and then serve.

Easy Veggie Egg Scramble

Scrambled eggs accompanied by a variety of strong vegetables and spices.

Prep time: 5 minutes

Cook time: 3-6 minutes

INGREDIENTS

2 cage-free eggs

1 small onion

1 clove garlic

½ red bell pepper

1 tbsp extra virgin olive oil

¼ tsp smoked paprika

¼ tsp ground black pepper

INSTRUCTIONS

1. Finely chop onion, garlic and red bell pepper.

2. Pour extra virgin olive oil into a pan over medium heat.

3. Crack eggs and pour into a small bowl. Combine with onion, garlic and red bell pepper and whisk until mixed together.

4. Pour contents of bowl into pan and add smoked paprika and ground black pepper. Scramble until desired doneness.

5. Serve.

Avocado Cream Blast

Tuna in a creamy avocado paste with red and blue fruit on the side.

Prep time: 3 minutes

INGREDIENTS

3 oz tuna

½ avocado

¼ tsp ground black pepper

½ cup blueberries

½ cup strawberries

INSTRUCTIONS

1. Mix tuna and avocado into a paste. Add ground black pepper and combine.
2. Chop strawberries and add them into blueberries.
3. Place both tuna and fruit mixtures on a plate and serve.

Spicy Egg Dish

Spicy scrambled eggs.

Prep time: 1 minute

Cook time: 3-6 minutes

INGREDIENTS

2 cage-free eggs

¼ tsp Celtic sea salt

¼ tsp curry powder

¼ tsp chipotle chili pepper powder

1 tbsp olive oil

INSTRUCTIONS

1. Over medium heat, pour olive oil into pan. Crack eggs and pour them into the pan. Combine seasonings and mix until desired doneness.

2. Serve.

Bell Pepper Fruit Cup

Turn a bell pepper into two bowls bursting with fresh fruity flavor in this alternative cereal-style recipe.

Prep time: 3 minutes

INGREDIENTS

1 bell pepper

1 cup coconut milk

1 banana

½ cup strawberries

½ cup blueberries

1 tsp cinnamon

INSTRUCTIONS

1. Slice bell pepper in half horizontally and place the pieces on a plate open-side up. Remove the seeds and fleshy interior walling. Slice the banana into small pieces.

2. Pour ½ cup coconut milk and half the total fruit into each bell pepper. Add cinnamon.

3. Serve.

Green Baked Avocado

Baked avocado filled with eggs and topped with chives.

Prep time: 3 minutes

Cook time: 15-20 minutes

INGREDIENTS

1 avocado

2 cage-free eggs

⅛ tsp ground black pepper

2 tsp chives

INSTRUCTIONS

1. Preheat oven to 425 degrees.

2. Slice the avocado in half and remove the nut. Scoop out enough flesh from the center of each avocado to contain the contents of 1 egg.

3. Crack the eggs and dump them into the middle of each piece of avocado. Place them on a baking sheet and bake for 15-20 minutes.

4. Remove from oven. Season with pepper and chives and serve.

Baked Egg Muffins

Baked egg muffins mixed with peppers and onion.

Prep time: 5 minutes

Cook time: 15-20 minutes

INGREDIENTS

1 tbsp olive oil

1 tbsp coconut oil

6 cage-free eggs

1 onion

½ yellow bell pepper

½ red bell pepper

¼ tsp ground black pepper

¼ tsp Celtic sea salt

INSTRUCTIONS

1. Preheat oven to 350. Whisk all 6 eggs in a bowl. Chop the onion and bell pepper into small pieces.

2. In a pan, combine olive oil with onion over medium-high heat for 2 minutes. Add peppers and cook another 2 minutes.

3. Remove onion/peppers from heat and let cool a few minutes. Combine them with the eggs. Add the Celtic sea salt and ground black pepper and mix.

4. Coat a muffin pan with the coconut oil. Fill each muffin cup with the egg/pepper/onion mix. Do not fill a muffin cup more than ¾ full.

5. Place the pan in the oven and bake 10-15 minutes, removing the pan from the oven when the tops of the muffins get fluffy and golden brown.

6. Remove the muffins from the pan and serve.

Spicy Chicken Wraps

Thinly sliced chicken meat wrapped around vegetables in an avocado paste.

Prep time: 5 minutes

Cook time: 3 minutes

INGREDIENTS

4 slices of chicken deli meat

1 tbsp olive oil

1 small onion

1 red bell pepper

1 avocado

¼ tsp garlic powder

INSTRUCTIONS

1. Remove the nut from the avocado and mash it into a paste. Chop the pepper and onion into small pieces.

2. Combine the garlic powder, pepper and onion in the bowl with the avocado and mix well.

3. Add the olive oil in a pan over low heat and heat the chicken mildly, turning frequently, for 3 minutes.

4. Remove the chicken from heat and place ¼ of the
   avocado/pepper/onion mixture onto each piece.

5. Wrap the chicken up into tubes and serve.

Delicious Apple Smoothie

Smoothie full of fall flavors.

Prep time: 5 minutes

INGREDIENTS

1 apple (honeycrisp preferred)

4 figs

½ avocado

1 handful kale

1 tsp cinnamon

1 cup apple cider

1. Slice avocado in half and remove the nut. Slice the apple into small pieces. Wash the figs, cut them in half and remove the stems.
2. Combine all ingredients except for the kale into a blender. Blend them until pureed, then add kale and blend until pureed.

Sugar Free Fruit Salad

A variety of fruits mixed with nuts, raw honey and cinnamon.

Prep time: 5 minutes

INGREDIENTS

½ banana

1 apple

¼ cup blueberries

½ cup strawberries

¼ cup slivered almonds

1 tbsp raw unfiltered honey

½ tsp cinnamon

INSTRUCTIONS

1. Slice banana, peel core and chop apple, slice strawberries.

2. Combine the fruit in a bowl with slivered almonds. Drizzle with honey and add cinnamon.

3. Serve.

Berry Cereal

A hot cereal of nuts and seeds accompanied by blueberries and coconut milk.

Prep time: overnight

Cook time: 1-2 minutes

INGREDIENTS

¼ cup sunflower seeds

¼ cup buckwheat

¼ cup pumpkin seeds

¼ cup flax seeds

¼ cup almonds

¼ cup blueberries

½ cup coconut milk

½ tsp cinnamon

INSTRUCTIONS

1. Combine sunflower seeds, buckwheat, pumpkin seeds, flax seeds and almonds in a bowl with water; this is done to sprout the seeds. Place the bowl in the fridge overnight.

2. In the morning drain the water from the bowl. Microwave the contents on high for 1-2 minutes to desired heat. Pour coconut milk into the bowl, mix, and top with blueberries and cinnamon. If desired, pour the coconut milk in before microwaving.

3. Serve.

Tahini with Fruit Topping

Celery stick slathered in cinnamon tahini and topped with fruits.

Prep time: 4 minutes

INGREDIENTS

1 large celery stalk

¼ cup tahini

2 tsp cinnamon

½ cup blueberries

½ cup strawberries

INSTRUCTIONS

1. In a small bowl, mix the cinnamon into the tahini. Wash the celery stalk and dry the concave inside. Chop the strawberries.

2. Spread the tahini mixture throughout the concave inside.

3. Stick the fruit into the tahini side by side alternating blueberry/strawberry.

4. Serve.

Sweet Potato Crisps with Eggs

Scrambled eggs and sweet potato fries.

Prep time: 4 minutes

Cook time: 10 minutes

INGREDIENTS

2 cage-free eggs

1 sweet potato

2 tbsp olive oil

¼ tsp Celtic sea salt

¼ tsp ground black pepper

¼ tsp oregano

INSTRUCTIONS

1. Slice the sweet potato into sticks. Combine in a pan with 1 tbsp olive oil and cook on medium-high heat, turning frequently, until browned, about 10 minutes depending on thickness of pieces.

2. In a separate pan crack the eggs and combine with 1 tbsp olive oil and scramble until desired done-ness.

3. On a plate, scatter the eggs and potato sticks. Season with Celtic sea salt, ground black pepper and oregano.

4. Serve.

Spicy Kale with Poached Eggs

Flavored kale topped with poached eggs and horseradish.

Prep time: 10 minutes

Cook time: 12 minutes

INGREDIENTS

1 handful kale

2 cage-free eggs

1 small onion

1 clove garlic

1 tbsp extra virgin olive oil

¼ tsp ground black pepper

1 tsp low-sodium horseradish (optional)

INSTRUCTIONS

1. Chop the onion and mince the garlic. De-stem and wash the kale. Leaving a bit of water on the kale is ideal.

2. In a saucepan, add 1 tbsp extra virgin olive oil over medium heat. Add onion and cook until it begins to lose its opaqueness, about 5 minutes.

3. Add kale to saucepan and cover until kale is soft and green, about 5 minutes. Add garlic and stir, then cook another 2 minutes and remove from heat.

4. Fill a saucepan half full of water. Bring the water to a boil, then reduce heat below a boil and hold it there.

5. One by one, crack the eggs into a small cup or bowl and, with the lip of the cup or bowl close to the water's surface, dump the egg into the water. If necessary, nudge the eggwhites closer to the yolks to keep them together.

6. Once all the eggs are in the water, remove the pan from heat and cover it. Let sit for 4 minutes until all eggs are cooked, then remove eggs from pan.

7. Place the greens on a plate and the two eggs on top of the greens. Top with horseradish if desired. Serve.

Wheat Free Pancakes with Berry Topping

Delicious paleo pancake wedges separated by a layer of red fruit sauce and topped with honey and strawberries.

Prep time: 10 minutes

Cook time: 20-25 minutes

INGREDIENTS

Pancake

½ cup organic almond butter

½ cup organic applesauce

2 cage-free eggs

¼ tsp cinnamon

Fruit dressing

2 stalks rhubarb

2 cups strawberries

¼ cup water

Toppings

whole strawberries

raw, unfiltered honey

INSTRUCTIONS

1. Chop the rhubarb and slice the strawberries. Place water, rhubarb and strawberries in a saucepan and simmer, covered, for 15 minutes.

2. Remove from heat and mash into a paste, then set aside.

3. Mix almond butter, applesauce, cinnamon and eggs in a bowl. Pour a thin layer of this into a frying pan over medium heat. Flip as you would a pancake and cook until thickened, about 1 to 2 minutes on each side. Set this pancake aside, recoat the bottom of the frying pan with another layer of the mixture, and cook this the same way.

4. Place the first pancake on a plate. Spread the fruit mixture over the surface of this pancake. Place the second pancake on top. Cut the breakfast cake across its diameter into 8 slices.

5. When serving a slice, drizzle with honey and top with 2 strawberries.

Sugar Free Baked Apples

Baked apples infused with lemon, raisin, cinnamon, ginger and nuts.

Prep time: 10 minutes

Cook time: 20-25 minutes

INGREDIENTS

3 apples

¼ cup raisins

¼ cup chopped almonds (or walnuts)

½ cup water

1 tbsp lemon juice

½ tsp cinnamon

¼ tsp ginger

raw, unfiltered honey

INSTRUCTIONS

1. Preheat oven to 350 degrees.

2. Slice and core apples. Place in an 8x8 baking pan. Pour water and lemon juice over the apples and let sit in baking dish. Sprinkle

raisins, almonds/walnuts, ginger and cinnamon over the top. Cover with tin foil and bake for 20-25 minutes or until apple is tender.

3. Remove from oven and serve in a bowl with honey drizzled over the top.

Very Berry Fruit Cereal

Hot liquidless cereal in a mixed berry sauce and topped with pomegranate seeds.

Prep time: 10 minutes

Cook time: 15 minutes

INGREDIENTS

¼ cup black raspberry

¼ cup raspberry

¼ cup blueberry

¼ cup strawberry

¼ cup water

1 cup buckwheat

1 pomegranate

INSTRUCTIONS:

1. Combine black raspberry, raspberry, blueberry, strawberry and ¼ cup water in a saucepan. Simmer, covered, and stirring occasionally, for 10 minutes.

2. Cook buckwheat according to package directions.

3. Remove seeds from pomegranate, and set seeds in a dish.

4. Spoon some buckwheat into a bowl. Scoop hot berry mixture over the top. Sprinkle pomegranate seeds over the top and serve.

Chopped Spicy Zucchini

Spinach, zucchini, yellow squash, garlic and thyme in a cage-free frittata.

Prep time: 10 minutes

Cook time: 15 minutes

INGREDIENTS

6 cage-free eggs

2 handfuls spinach

2 cloves garlic

1 small zucchini

1 small yellow squash

1 tbsp extra virgin olive oil

¼ tsp Celtic sea salt

¼ tsp ground black pepper

¼ tsp thyme

INSTRUCTIONS

1. Crack eggs into a bowl and mix them with thyme. Mince garlic, chop zucchini and yellow squash half-moon slices.

2. Heat oil in a frying pan over medium heat. Saute garlic, zucchini and yellow squash for 4 minutes, stirring occasionally.

3. Add spinach and wilt, covered, for 1 minute.

4. Pour eggs over top, cover, and reduce to low heat. Cook through, about 10 minutes. Remove from pan and sprinkle Celtic sea salt and ground black pepper over the top.

Lunch Cookbook

Squash with Sliced Mushroom

Prep time: 15-20 minutes

Cook time: approx 20 minutes

Serves: 2

INGREDIENTS

1 large yellow squash

½ pound organic grass-fed ground turkey

2 tbsp extra virgin olive oil

4 baby portobella mushrooms

2 cloves garlic

2 small tomatoes

12 leaves fresh basil

12 oz organic additive-free tomato sauce

3 oz olive tapenade

INSTRUCTIONS

1. Mince the garlic and cut the yellow squash into 12 slices. Cut tomatoes into 12 slices. Slice mushrooms into 12 total slices.

2. Sautee ½ pound ground turkey in 1 tbsp extra virgin olive oil in a saucepan until no longer pink. Then add minced garlic and sautee 2-3 minutes.

3. Add 12 oz organic additive-free tomato sauce and sautee until it bubbles. Remove from heat.

4. Sautee sliced mushrooms in a pan with 1 tbsp extra virgin olive oil until light brown, about 2-3 minutes.

5. For each slice of yellow squash, layer with olive tapenade, then tomato, then meat sauce, then mushroom, then basil. Serve.

Zucchini Onion Rolls

Prep time: 15 minutes

Cook time: 10 minutes

Serves: 2

INGREDIENTS

1 large zucchini

2-3 cloves garlic

6.5 oz artichoke hearts

½ medium onion

6 slices low sodium organic grass-fed turkey bacon

12 oz organic additive-free tomato sauce

½ green pepper

¼ tsp dried basil

¼ tsp dried oregano

¼ tsp ground black pepper

INSTRUCTIONS

1. Cut zucchini lengthwise into 8 pliable sheets. Mince the garlic and dice the onion, green pepper and artichoke.

2. Sautee bacon until it's browned. Remove the bacon from the pan and crumble. Set aside.

3. Put green pepper and onion in the pan and sautee for 2 minutes. Add garlic and sautee for another minute. Add artichoke and red sauce and bring to a bubble, about 5 minutes.

4. Add crumbled bacon and dried basil, oregano and ground black pepper to the pan. Thoroughly stir together.

5. For each slice of zucchini, spread cooked mixture evenly across the top and then roll up. Serve.

Avocado & Tomato Pizza

Prep time: 7 minutes

Cook time: 3-4 minutes

Serves: 2

INGREDIENTS

2 avocados

2 low sodium organic grass-fed turkey sauce links (pre-cooked)

½ cup chopped pineapple

1 large tomato

1 tbsp extra virgin olive oil

INSTRUCTIONS

1. Slice avocados in half. Remove the pit and the peel and set aside.

2. Dice the sausage and tomato into small pieces and add into a pan with extra virgin olive oil along with chopped pineapple. Heat through, about 3-4 minutes.

3. Place two halves of avocado on 1 plate each. Evenly distribute the sauteed ingredients into each avocado. Drizzle the remaining mixture over each avocado. Serve.

Red & Yellow Pepper Pizza

Prep time: 15 minutes

Cook time: 15 minutes

Serves: 2

INGREDIENTS

Pizza

1 red pepper

1 yellow pepper

1 small red onion

1 low-sodium cooked organic grass-fed chicken sausage link

1 cup broccoli florets

1 tbsp extra virgin olive oil

Pesto

1 packed cup fresh basil

¼ cup extra virgin olive oil

¼ cup walnuts

3 cloves garlic

¼ tsp Celtic sea salt

¼ tsp ground black pepper

INSTRUCTIONS

1. Cut the peppers in half. Remove the stems, cores and seeds. Line a baking sheet with aluminum foil and place the peppers in it skin side up. Put peppers under the broiler and leave them there until the skin has begun to turn black and shriveled.

2. Remove peppers from oven, place in a plastic bag and place in refrigerator until cool.

3. Peel the skins off the peppers and throw them away.

4. Slice the onion into half moon slices and slice the chicken sausage link into twelve thin slices. Place the onion, sausage slices and broccoli florets with 1 tbsp extra virgin olive oil in a saucepan over medium heat for 4 minutes until vegetables are tender crisp and meat is slightly browned.

5. Place all the pesto ingredients in a food processor and blend until smooth.

6. Put two halves of roasted pepper on a dish, one red and one yellow, open side up. Using a spoon, spread pesto evenly inside each pepper half. Evenly distribute broccoli, onion, and sausage over the tops.

7. Serve.

Easy Spicy Eggplant Dish

Prep time: 10 minutes

Cook time: 8 minutes

Serves: 2

INGREDIENTS

½ large eggplant cut lengthwise

4 asparagus stalks

2 cloves garlic

1 yellow tomato

2 tsp fresh cilantro

2 tbsp extra virgin olive oil

1 cup organic red sauce

INSTRUCTIONS

1. In a medium saucepan, heat the red sauce on low and keep hot.

2. Slice the eggplant into ½ inch slices, 8 slices total. Heat 1 ½ extra virgin olive oil in a frying pan on medium heat. Cook the eggplant two minutes on one side and another two minutes on the other side. Transfer to a plate.

3. Add ½ tbsp to the pan. Slice the garlic. Rinse the asparagus and cut each asparagus stalk into 3 equal lengths.

4. Add garlic and asparagus to pan and sautee until asparagus is tender.

5. Dice yellow tomato and cilantro and mix together.

6. Place four slices of eggplant on each plate. Spoon red sauce over each slice. Cover with tomato/cilantro mixture and evenly distribute asparagus and garlic cloves.

7. Serve.

Nutty Harvest Boat

Prep time: 10 minutes

Cook time: 6-8 minutes

Serves: 2

INGREDIENTS

2 delicata squash

6 oz bag of organic coleslaw mix

3 scallions

1 cup slivered almonds

¼ cup sunflower seeds

1 medium carrot

1 mandarin orange

2 celery stalks

2 tbsp raw unfiltered honey

2 tbsp vinegar

¼ cup extra virgin olive oil

INSTRUCTIONS

1. Chop the scallions and celery and shred the carrot. Peel the orange.

   Cut the delicata squash in half lengthwise and dispose of the seeds.

2. Place the squash in a microwave safe dish cut side up. Put 1 tbsp of water in the bottom of the dish. Cover and microwave on high for 6 minutes. Test with fork and if the fork doesn't go in easily, continue microwaving until it does.

3. In a medium sized mixing bowl, placing the larger ingredients in first, combine scallions, slivered almonds, sunflower seeds, carrot, orange slices and celery. Mix well.

4. In a small bowl, mix the honey, vinegar and extra virgin olive oil. Pour this mixture over the other ingredients and mix.

5. Scoop this mixture evenly into each half of delicata squash. Place two halves on each plate.

6. Serve.

Cucumber Raft

Prep time: 20 minutes

Cook time: 15 minutes

Serves: 2

INGREDIENTS

2 cucumbers

2 cups shredded lettuce

1 medium sized tomato

1 cup cooked quinoa

½ avocado

½ cup grapes

¼ cup chopped walnuts

2 tbsp raspberry vinaigrette

INSTRUCTIONS

1. Peel the cucumbers and cut in half lengthwise. Scoop out seeds and discard. Dice the tomato and avocado and cut the grapes in half.

2. Put ¼ cup of the cooked quinoa inside the hollow core of each slice of cucumber. Then distribute the following ingredients evenly across each cucumber in the following order: shredded lettuce,

tomato, avocado, grapes and chopped walnuts. Drizzle the raspberry vinaigrette over the tops of each.

3. Serve.

Ratatouille Riverboat

Prep time: 10 minutes

Cook time: 1 hour

Serves: 2

INGREDIENTS

1 large eggplant

1 medium zucchini

½ onion

1 cup mushrooms

½ green bell pepper

1 tomato

1 cup vegetable stock

2 cloves garlic

2 tbsp extra virgin olive oil

½ tsp thyme

¼ tsp parsley

INSTRUCTIONS

1. Preheat oven to 400 degrees.

2. Cut the eggplant in half lengthwise and scoop out the seeds, leaving an oblong bowl through the middle of each. Brush with 1 tbsp extra virgin olive oil. Place them cut side down on a baking sheet lined with parchment paper. Place in the oven for one hour.

3. Chop the green bell pepper, tomato, zucchini and onion. Slice the mushrooms. Combine all these ingredients in a medium saucepan with 1 tbsp extra virgin olive oil. Saute over medium heat for 4 minutes.

4. Add vegetable stock, thyme and parsley to the saucepan and let simmer until some of the liquid cooks down, approximately 10 minutes.

5. Place each half of eggplant on a plate and scoop out the vegetable mixture over the top of each.

Fruitychicken Melonboat

Prep time: 20 minutes

Cook time: 10 minutes

Serves: 2

INGREDIENTS

1 small watermelon

½ cup black raspberries

½ cup Juan canary melon

1 organic grass-fed chicken breast

1 shallot

2 clementines

½ green pepper

1 tbsp extra virgin olive oil

INSTRUCTIONS

1. Cube the Juan canary melon. Peel the clementine and divide into wedges. Chop the green pepper and shallot. Cut the watermelon in half, scoop out the flesh and chop it up. Set rind aside.

2. Grill the chicken for 2-3 minutes on each side until no longer pink. Chop the chicken into cubes and set aside.

3. In a small pan, combine extra virgin olive oil, chopped pepper and shallot. Sautee for 4 minutes.

4. Place all the ingredients in a medium bowl and mix evenly with a spoon. Scoop half the ingredients into each watermelon bowl. Serve.

Barreling Down the River

Prep time: 10 minutes

Cook time: 15 minutes

Serves: 2

INGREDIENTS

2 red bell peppers

1 green bell pepper

1 filet of haddock

1 medium onion

1 medium tomato

1 can organic tomato paste

½ tsp oregano

¼ tsp Celtic sea salt

¼ tsp ground black pepper

2 tbsp extra virgin olive oil

INSTRUCTIONS

1. Chop the tops off the red bell peppers and core them, removing the seeds and white fleshy interior. Set aside. Chop the green bell pepper and onion. Dice the tomato.

2. In a medium saucepan heat the green bell pepper and onion in extra virgin olive oil over medium heat for 4 minutes. Add the tomato and the can of tomato paste, stir and let simmer for another 5 minutes.

3. In a frying pan, heat 1 tbsp extra virgin olive oil over medium heat and add the fish filet. Cook until the fish flakes easily, about 5-7 minutes, turning once.

4. Add the filet to the saucepan with all remaining ingredients and seasonings, stirring the ingredients together and breaking up the filet into smaller pieces.

5. Scoop the contents into the bell peppers and serve, one on each plate.

Red Wrap

Prep time: 20 minutes

Serves: 2

INGREDIENTS

Wrap

6 slices organic grass-fed deli turkey

½ red bell pepper

6 cherry tomatoes

½ avocado

6 arugula leaves

Pesto

½ packed cup fresh basil

2 tbsp extra virgin olive oil

2 tbsp almonds

1 clove garlic

¼ tsp Celtic sea salt

INSTRUCTIONS

1. Chop the red bell pepper. Mash the avocado.

2. Combine the pesto ingredients in a food processor and puree. Set aside.

3. Stack 3 slices of turkey and spread half the pesto across the top. Across the middle, lay ¼ cup chopped red bell pepper, half the avocado mash, 3 cherry tomatoes and 3 arugula leaves. Repeat this process for the other 3 slices of turkey and wrap them both up, securing with toothpicks. Serve.

Spicy Seafruit Wraps

Prep time: 15 minutes

Serves: 2

INGREDIENTS

4 sheets of Nori

1 can of tuna fish

1 tbsp extra virgin olive oil

1 tsp dried mustard

2 scallions

¼ cup raspberry

1 tbsp raw unfiltered honey

INSTRUCTIONS

1. Moisten the Nori to make it pliable. Chop the scallions.

2. Combine the tuna, extra virgin olive oil, dried mustard and chopped scallions and mix them together into a blend.

3. Spread the blend into each piece of Nori and wrap them up. Drizzle with honey and place raspberries on top. Serve.

Dragonchicken Wraps

Prep time: 15 minutes

Serves: 2

INGREDIENTS

6 slices organic grass-fed deli chicken

1 jalapeno

2 stalks celery

½ avocado

1 tbsp fresh basil

INSTRUCTIONS

1. Chop the jalapeno pepper and mash the avocado. Slice the celery into stalks that fit the diameter of a slice of deli chicken meat.

2. Stack 3 slices of deli chicken and spread the avocado mash across the middle. Place the celery through the center, sprinkle the basil across the middle and then evenly distribute the jalapeno slices. Wrap the chicken up and secure with toothpicks. Save enough of each ingredient to repeat this process across the other 3 slices of deli chicken. Serve.

Eggplant Chicken Burgers

Prep time: 15 minutes

Cook time: 8 minutes

Serves: 2

INGREDIENTS

Burger

1 eggplant

4 small organic grass-fed chicken breasts or thighs

1 tomato

1 onion

1 handful romaine lettuce

1 tbsp coconut oil

¼ tsp smoked paprika

Sauce

¼ packed cup fresh basil

2 tbsp extra virgin olive oil

1 clove garlic

2 tbsp walnuts

¼ tsp Celtic sea salt

INSTRUCTIONS

1. Combine the sauce ingredients in a food processor and puree.

2. Slice the eggplant into 8 round slices. Slice the tomato and onion into 4 slices each. Break the romaine lettuce up into smaller pieces.

3. Sprinkle the chicken with smoked paprika and combine with coconut oil in a small pan over medium heat. Sautee until cooked through and no longer pink, about 4 minutes on each side.

4. Assemble 4 burgers in the following manner: 1 slice eggplant, 1 piece chicken, 1 slice tomato, 1 slice onion, drizzled sauce, 1 slice eggplant. Secure with toothpick if desired. Serve 2 burgers to each person.

Chickenfish Wraps

Prep time:

Serves: 2

INGREDIENTS

6 slices organic grass-fed deli chicken

1 can tuna

2 tbsp extra virgin olive oil

½ tsp smoked paprika

½ avocado

INSTRUCTIONS

1. Mix tuna, extra virgin olive oil, smoked paprika and avocado into a paste.

2. Stack 3 slices of deli chicken and spread the paste across the diameter of the top. Wrap the chicken up and secure with toothpicks. Repeat for the other 3 slices and serve.

Mangospice Chicken Soup

Prep time: 15 minutes

Cook time: 45 minutes

Serves: 2

INGREDIENTS

2 cups organic vegetable stock

2 organic grass-fed chicken breasts

1 red bell pepper

1 yellow bell pepper

½ onion

1 clove garlic

1 cup mango

1 tbsp extra virgin olive oil

2 tbsp lemon juice

¼ tsp Celtic sea salt

¼ tsp ground black pepper

INSTRUCTIONS

1. Cut the peppers in half. Remove the stems, cores and seeds. Line a baking sheet with aluminum foil and place the peppers in it skin

side up. Put peppers under the broiler and leave them there until the skin has begun to turn black and shriveled.

2. Remove peppers from oven, place in a plastic bag and place in refrigerator until cool.

3. Peel the skins off the peppers and throw them away. Chop the peppers.

4. Preheat oven to 350. Place chicken on a baking dish with extra virgin olive oil and lemon juice. Bake for 20 minutes or until chicken is no longer pink.

5. Chop the onion and mango and crush the garlic.

6. Place onion and garlic in a large saucepan with ½ cup vegetable stock and boil for 5 minutes. Add the rest of the stock and the roasted peppers and bring it back to a boil. Turn the heat down, cover, and let simmer for 5 minutes.

7. Using an immersion blender, blend the contents of the saucepan. Chop up the cooked chicken and place it, along with the mango, in the saucepan.

8. Season with sea salt and ground black pepper and heat through.

9. Serve.

Earthroot Soup

Prep time: 5 minutes

Cook time: 15 minutes

Serves: 2

INGREDIENTS

½ quart organic vegetable stock

½ leek

1 cup celery root

3 oz fresh spinach

1 cup cauilfllower

¼ tsp Celtic sea salt

¼ tsp ground black pepper

¼ tsp nutmeg

1 ½ tsp grated fresh ginger

INSTRUCTIONS

1. Slice the leek and dice the celery root. Cut the cauliflower into florets.

2. Pour the vegetable stock in a saucepan and add the leeks, celery root, cauliflower florets, ginger and spinach. Bring to a boil.

Reduce heat and simmer for 10-15 minutes until vegetables are tender.

3. Using an immersion blender, blend the contents of the saucepan until pureed.

4. Season with Celtic sea salt, ground black pepper and nutmeg.

5. Serve.

Omelet Soup

Prep time: 5 minutes

Cook time: 18-20 minutes

Serves: 2

INGREDIENTS

1 oz organic grass-fed turkey bacon

2 cage-free eggs

½ onion

1 tbsp extra virgin olive oil

6 oz portabella mushrooms

1 ½ cups organic chicken stock

2 tsp Italian seasoning

2 springs of sage

¼ tsp Celtic sea salt

¼ tsp ground black pepper

INSTRUCTIONS

1. Chop the onion. Roughly chop the bacon and place it in a medium saucepan on medium heat. Cook through.

2. Add the onion and extra virgin olive oil and stir. Chop the mushrooms and add to the pan. Cover and cook for 2-3 minutes.

3. Add the chicken stock, seasoning, Celtic sea salt and ground black pepper to taste. Cover and simmer for 10 minutes.

4. Using an egg poacher if available, poach both eggs in the soup.

5. Serve and garnish with sage.

Trail Mix Soup

Prep time: 5-10 minutes

Cook time: 25-30 minutes

Serves 2:

INGREDIENTS

2 cups organic vegetable stock

1 oz coconut milk

½ red onion

1 heaping cup chopped sweet potato

1 apple

½ tsp ginger powder

2 tbsp extra virgin olive oil

¼ tsp cinnamon

1 tbsp chopped scallion

1 tbsp slivered almonds

¼ tsp Celtic sea salt

¼ tsp ground black pepper

2 tsp shredded coconut

INSTRUCTIONS

1. Mince the onion and slice and chop the apple.

2. In a medium saucepan, combine extra virgin olive oil and onion and cook over medium heat for 5 minutes.

3. Add sweet potato and apple and sautee for another 3 minutes.

4. Mix in ginger, cinnamon, scallion, Celtic sea salt and ground black pepper. Reduce heat to lowand sautee another 10 minutes, stirring occasionally.

5. Add vegetable stock and almonds and stir. Cover and simmer for 8-10 minutes until vegetables are soft.

6. Add coconut milk to soup and stir well.

7. Serve and garnish with shredded coconut.

Honeyfruit Soup

Prep time: 15 minutes

Serves: 2

INGREDIENTS

1 cantaloupe

1 cup sliced cooked beets

½ cup water

1 lime

1 tbsp shredded basil

basil leaves for garnishing

raw, organic honey for garnishing

INSTRUCTIONS

1. Slice the beets. Scrape out any seeds in the melon and throw away. Squeeze the juice out of the lime.

2. Using a melon baller scoop ten balls out of the cantaloupe. Leave at least one half of the cantaloupe untouched. Set aside for garnish.

3. Scoop out the rest of the cantaloupe and place in a blender or food processor. Add water, beets and lime juice and blend.

4. Transfer the mixture to a bowl, add the shredded basil and stir. Place in the refrigerator to chill for at least 30 minutes.

5. When serving, add 5 cantaloupe balls to each bowl and garnish with basil leaves and drizzle with honey.

Dinner Cookbook

Lemon Chicken & Vegetable Blend

Prep time: 4 minutes

Cook time: 8 minutes

Servings: 4

INGREDIENTS

4 pieces grass-fed chicken thighs

1 onion

2 cloves garlic

3/4 cup sliced carrots

2 handfuls Kale greens

2 tbsp chinese five spice

2 tbsp smoked paprika

2 tbsp chipotle chili pepper powder

1 tbsp olive oil

2 tsp lemon juice

1 tbsp coconut oil

INSTRUCTIONS

1. Mince garlic and chop onion to desired size (medium strips work

    best). Chop carrots to 1/4" thickness. De-rib the kale and chop it coarsely, wash it and allow water to remain on the leaves. Bring 4 cups of water to a light boil.

2. Heat 1 tbsp olive oil over medium heat in a large pan. Add carrot and onion and cook for 8 minutes, stirring occasionally.

3. Meanwhile, heat 1 tbsp coconut oil over medium heat in a separate pan. Add chicken and cook for 4 minutes. Season chicken with chinese five spice, chipotle chili pepper powder and smoked paprika and turn, adding more of each spice to the other side of the chicken, cooking for another 4 minutes or until cooked through.

4. Add kale to boiling water and boil until bright green, about 5 minutes. Remove from water and let sit while the vegetables and chicken continue cooking.

5. Add everything into the pan with the vegetables and add 2 tsp lemon juice. Add minced garlic and stir for 1 minute.

6. Serve immediately.

Chopped Chicken & Veggie Salad

Prep time: 24 hours (date syrup is created overnight)

Cook time: 50 minutes

Servings: 4

INGREDIENTS

Date Syrup

1 cup water

1 cup pitted dates

Salad

4 pieces grass-fed chicken thighs, coarsely chopped

1 tbsp extra virgin olive oil

7 oz bag Romaine lettuce

1 red bell pepper

1 yellow bell pepper

½ cup walnuts

1 cup strawberries

1 cup kiwi

INSTRUCTIONS

1. For Date Syrup, split the dates down the middle, remove the pits, and place in a bowl with 1 cup water. Place this mixture in the fridge overnight. Stir occasionally if you are able to.

2. Preheat oven to 375. Take the chopped chicken thighs and coat them in olive oil. Place them on a baking dish, cover with aluminum foil, and place them in the oven for 30 minutes.

3. Chop the peppers and slice the strawberries and kiwi.

4. When the chicken has cooked for 30 minutes, remove the aluminum foil and cook for another 15 minutes. After 15 minutes, drizzle half the date syrup mixture over the chicken and cook another 5 minutes.

5. Place the romaine lettuce, peppers, walnuts, strawberries and kiwis in a bowl and toss.

6. Remove chicken from oven and place into the bowl. Drizzle the remaining date syrup over the finished dish and toss.

7. Serve immediately or chill 20 minutes and serve.

Delicious Baked Juicy Meat

Prep time: 10 minutes

Cook time: 25 minutes

Serves: 4

INGREDIENTS

4 pieces grass-fed chicken thighs

4 cloves garlic

4 stems rosemary

3 tbsp extra-virgin olive oil

1 lemon

¼ tsp ground black pepper

½ cup organic chicken stock

INSTRUCTIONS

1. Preheat oven to 450 degrees.

2. Strip the leaves from the rosemary and crush the garlic. Grate the lemon into zest and juice and separate the two.

3. Place chicken on a baking dish. Add garlic, rosemary, lemon zest, olive oil and ground black pepper. Toss chicken to coat thoroughly and roast (uncovered) 20 minutes.

4. After 20 minutes of roasting, add chicken broth and lemon juice. Turn over chicken.

5. Return to oven, turn oven off and let sit 5 minutes longer.

6. Remove from oven and place on serving dish, pouring pan juices over the chicken. Serve immediately or chill 20 minutes and serve.

Spicy Stewed Steaks

Prep time: 10 minutes

Cook time: 6 minutes

Serves: 4

INGREDIENTS

3 lbs. Swordfish steak

¾ cup parsley leaves

1 clove garlic

¼ tsp Celtic sea salt

2 lemons

extra virgin olive oil

6 tomatoes

1 onion

4 cups chopped arugula

ground black pepper (to taste)

INSTRUCTIONS

1. Preheat broiler. Grate the zest from one lemon. Seed and chop
    tomatoes and chop the onion, and combine with arugula. Drizzle
    with extra virgin olive oil and season with Celtic sea salt and

ground black pepper. Set the salad aside to be served equally over 4 plates.

2. Cut swordfish into 1-inch cubes and push onto 4 skewers.

3. Combine lemon zest, parsley and garlic and chop together. Add Celtic sea salt into the mixture and rub it in with the flat of your knife until it forms a paste.

4. Drizzle fish with extra virgin olive oil and rub the paste into the kebabs.

5. Place kebabs on broiler pan and broil on top rack until the fish is firm and opaque, approx. 3 minutes on each side.

6. Place 1 skewer on each of the 4 plates, on top of the salad. Serve immediately or chill 20 minutes and then serve.

Oven Cooked Vegetable & Stew Blend

Prep time: 15 minutes

Cook time: 3 hr 45 minutes

Serves: 6

INGREDIENTS

1 ½ lbs beef stew meat

1 onion

1 (14.5 oz) can no-salt added stewed tomatoes, undrained

¼ tsp Celtic sea salt

½ tsp ground black pepper

1 dried bay leaf

2 cups water

3 tbsp arrowroot powder

12 small sweet potatoes cut in half

30 baby-cut carrots

INSTRUCTIONS

1. Heat oven to 325 degrees. In a bowl, mix arrowroot in water and stir to a paste (if you're not using arrowroot, use 1 cup water instead). Cut the onion into 8 wedges and cut potatoes in half.

2. In ovenproof Dutch oven, mix beef, onion, tomatoes, Celtic sea salt, ground black pepper and bay leaf. Mix arrowroot-thickened water (or 1 cup water) into Dutch oven.

3. Cover and bake for 2 hours, stirring one time.

4. Stir in the potatoes and carrots. Cover and bake until beef and vegetables are tender, about 1 hr 45 min. Remove bay leaf and serve immediately, or chill 20 minutes and then serve.

Mirepoix with Red Sauce

Prep time: 7 minutes

Cook time: approx. 15 minutes

Serves: 4

INGREDIENTS

Flounder and Mirepoix

4 flounder fillets

1 tbsp extra virgin olive oil

¼ tsp thyme

¼ tsp parsley

1 clove garlic

1 stalk celery

8 baby-cut carrots

1 small onion

¼ cup water

¼ cup clam juice

Roasted Red Pepper sauce

1 tbsp extra virgin olive oil

1/2 small onion

1 clove garlic

¼ tsp smoked paprika

¼ tsp Celtic sea salt

¼ tsp ground white pepper

2 roasted red peppers

3/4 cup organic chicken stock

1 tbsp arrowroot

INSTRUCTIONS

1. For Mirepoix, finely chop the celery, carrots and 1 onion together and place in a bowl.

2. For Roasted Red Pepper sauce, finely chop the ½ onion and combine all the above listed Roasted Red Pepper sauce ingredients together in a pan. Keep warm over very low heat.

3. Combine thyme, parsley and extra virgin olive oil in a braising pan over medium-high heat. Add mirepoix and cook while stirring for

2-3 min until the vegetables are soft but not browned. Add clam juice and Roasted Red Pepper sauce. Season to taste with Celtic sea salt and ground white pepper. Reduce heat to medium-low and simmer 5 min.

4. Season fillets with Celtic sea salt and ground white pepper. Fold the thin end of each fillet underneath itself and place in the pan. Increase heat to a moderate simmer. Cover and poach 5-7 min until internal temperature reaches 130 degrees.

5. Remove fillets from pan and let rest 2 min. Serve immediately afterward, or chill 20 minutes and then serve.

Quick Asian Veggie Soup

Prep time: 5 minutes

Cook time: approx 35 minutes

Serves: 4

INGREDIENTS

1 banana

1 onion

1 clove garlic

1 pinch nutmeg

1 ½ tbsp cinnamon

3 cups pumpkin

1 pint organic chicken stock

⅔ cup orange juice

2 tbsp extra virgin olive oil

2 tbsp sunflower seeds

¼ tsp Celtic sea salt

¼ tsp ground black pepper

INSTRUCTIONS

1. Seed, peel and cube the pumpkin.

2. Mash the banana, finely chop the onion and crush the clove of garlic. Add all three into a large saucepan with 1 tbsp extra virgin olive oil and fry gently 4-5 minutes, until soft.

3. Stir in spices and pumpkin and cook over medium heat for 6 minutes, stirring occasionally.

4. Pour in the chicken stock and orange juice. Cover and bring to a boil, then reduce heat and simmer for 20 minutes, until the pumpkin is soft.

5. Pour half the mixture into a blender or food processor and blend until smooth. Return the blended mixture to the pan and continue stirring. Add the Celtic sea salt, black pepper, cinnamon and nutmeg.

6. Add 1 tbsp extra virgin olive oil and sunflower seeds to a small pan and fry for 1-2 minutes.

7. Serve the soup immediately with the sunflower seeds over top, or chill 20 minutes and then serve.

Spicy Oregano Cubes

Prep time: 1 hr 10 minutes

Cook time: 16-20 minutes

Serves: 4

INGREDIENTS

1 boneless leg of lamb

5 tbsp extra virgin olive oil

2 tsp dried oregano

1 tbsp fresh parsley

1 lemon

½ eggplant

4 small onions

2 tomatoes

5 fresh bay leaves

¼ tsp Celtic sea salt

¼ tsp ground black pepper

INSTRUCTIONS

1. Cube the lamb, chop the fresh parsley, juice the lemon, slice and quarter the eggplant into thick pieces, halve the onions and quarter the tomatoes.

2. Place lamb in a bowl. Mix olive oil, oregano, parsley, lemon juice and Celtic sea salt and ground black pepper. Pour this over the lamb and mix well. Cover and marinate for 1 hour.

3. Preheat the grill. Thread the marinated lamb, eggplant, onions, tomatoes and bay leaves in evenly on each of four skewers.

4. Place the kebabs on a grill inside a grill pan and brush them evenly with the leftover marinade until the marinade is all gone. Cook over medium heat turning once the kebabs once, for about 8-10 minutes on each side, basting them whenever enough juice collects in the bottom of the grill pan.

5. Serve immediately or chill 20 minutes and then serve.

Lamb Slits

Prep time: 10 minutes

Cook time: 1 hr 30 min

Serves: 4

INGREDIENTS

1 half leg of lamb

1 tbsp oregano

¼ tsp cumin

¼ tsp chipotle chili powder

2 cloves garlic

2 tbsp extra virgin olive oil

2 tbsp red wine vinegar

½ lemon

½ tsp ground black pepper

INSTRUCTIONS

1. Preheat oven to 425 degrees.

2. Crush 1 clove of garlic. Combine oregano, cumin, chipotle chili powder and garlic in a bowl. Pour 1 tbsp extra virgin olive oil and mix well to form a paste.

3. With a knife, make a criss-cross pattern of ½" slits through the skin, cutting slightly through the meat. Press the spice paste into the meat slits with the back of the knife.

4. Mince the last clove of garlic. Again, push this clove deeply into the slits in the lamb.

5. Mix the red wine vinegar and ground black pepper with extra virgin olive oil and pour over the lamb.

6. Bake for 15 minutes and then reduce heat to 350 degrees and cook for 1 ¼ hours longer. This will yield medium-cooked meat.

7. Serve immediately with pan juices or chill 20 minutes and then serve.

Spicy Kale Quiche

Prep time: 10 minutes

Cook time: 15 minutes

Serves: 4

INGREDIENTS

8 cage-free eggs

2 tbsp extra virgin olive oil

1 7oz bag of Kale greens

1 shallot

¼ tsp chipotle chili pepper powder

2 cloves garlic

½ lemon

2 tbsp coconut oil

¼ tbsp ground black pepper

INSTRUCTIONS

1. Place a steamer basket in the bottom of a large pot and fill with water; if you see water rise above the bottom of the basket, pour some out. Bring the water to a boil.

2. Wash the kale and remove the stems. Mince the garlic and shallot and squeeze the juice from the lemon into a bowl.

3. In a large pan, add the eggs and extra virgin olive oil. Mixing in the chipotle chili pepper powder, scramble the eggs, breaking them up until they form many small pieces, tender yet firm.

4. Place the kale in the pot and steam until tender and bright-green.

5. Remove the kale from the pot and combine with the eggs. Add the garlic, shallot and lemon juice, drizzle the coconut oil over top and add the ground black pepper. Mix and stir thoroughly.

6. Serve immediately or chill 20 minutes and then serve.

Red Pepper Chicken Fries

Prep time: 10 minutes

Cook time: 12 minutes

Serves: 4

INGREDIENTS

4 pieces grass-fed chicken thighs

1 large red pepper

1 large yellow pepper

1 large orange pepper

1 onion

1 clove garlic

1 tbsp coconut oil

¼ tsp ground black pepper

¼ tsp chinese five spice

INSTRUCTIONS

1. Chop the chicken into small cubes, about 1" each. Chop the peppers and onion into ½" cubes. Mince garlic.

2. In a pan, combine coconut oil with peppers and onion and cook over medium heat for 4 minutes.

3. Add chicken, pepper, chinese five spice, and stir, cooking 4 more minutes.

4. Flip and mix well (in order to cook chicken evenly), add garlic, and cook for 4 more minutes, or until chicken is cooked through.

5. Serve immediately or chill 20 minutes and then serve.

Nuts & Turkey Burgers

Prep time: 10 minutes

Cook time: 6-12 minutes

Servings: 4

INGREDIENTS

16 oz ground turkey

1 cup walnuts

2 cloves garlic

1 onion

¼ tsp chipotle chili pepper powder

¼ tbsp smoked paprika

¼ tsp ground black pepper

INSTRUCTIONS

1. Chop walnuts into smaller pieces, about ⅛" cubes. Mince garlic and chop onion into small pieces, about ¼" pieces.

2. Combine the above with ground turkey and add chipotle chili pepper powder, smoked paprika and ground black pepper. Knead it all together and separate into four patties.

3. Cook on the grill on high heat, flipping occasionally, until desired done-ness.

Sugar Free Meat Drizzle

Prep time: 24 hours (date syrup is created overnight)

Cook time: 1 hr 25 minutes

Serves: 4

INGREDIENTS

Date Syrup

1 cup water

1 cup pitted dates

Entree

2 medium-large sweet potatoes

12 oz ground turkey

¼ tbsp smoked paprika

¼ tsp ground black pepper

¼ tbsp extra virgin olive oil

INSTRUCTIONS

1. For Date Syrup, split the dates down the middle, remove the pits, and place in a bowl with 1 cup water. Place this mixture in the fridge overnight. Stir occasionally if you are able to.

2. Preheat oven to 375. Wash potatoes and wrap in aluminum foil. Knead ground turkey with smoked paprika and ground black pepper.

3. Bake potatoes for 1 hour, turning once. Remove from oven, unwrap and let cool, then cut in half.

4. When the potatoes are removed from the oven, begin sauteing ground turkey in a large pan with extra virgin olive oil over medium high heat, breaking up into small pieces. Saute until cooked through, approx 10 minutes.

5. Hollow out the center of each of the 4 slices of potatoes. The size of the hollow should be enough to fit ⅛ of the total ground turkey, so that there is some ground turkey above the surface of the hollow. Do not add the ground turkey yet.

6. Drizzle ¼ of the date syrup mixture into the hollow of each sweet potato and across the tops of each. Add the ground beef and return to the oven at 350 degrees for 15 minutes.

7. Remove potatoes from the oven and let col 5 minutes. Serve afterward or chill 20 minutes and then serve.

Chickplant Filets

Prep time: 10 minutes

Cook time: 50 minutes

Serves: 4

INGREDIENTS

4 grass-fed chicken breasts

1 eggplant

4 pinches fresh basil

¼ tsp chipotle chili pepper powder

¼ tsp curry

1 large carrot

1 red onion

1 cup coconut milk

8 wooden toothpicks

1 tbsp coconut oil

INSTRUCTIONS

1. Cut eggplant into 8 rectangles 3" long by 1" wide and 1" tall. Cut the carrot into matchsticks and dice the onion into small pieces. Cut the chicken in half lengthwise into thin filets. Soak the toothpicks in water. Preheat oven to 350.

2. Combine coconut oil, carrot, onion, 1 tsp curry, basil and chipotle chili pepper powder in a pan over medium heat. Stir together until it forms a sauce. Add eggplant and saute 7-10 minutes or until eggplant is tender.

3. Place 1 slice of eggplant on each of the chicken filets. Drizzle the contents of the pan over each of the filets; roll each fillet up around the eggplant and secure with a toothpick.

4. Place the 8 filets in the oven and bake for 35 minutes.

5. Remove from oven and pour serve 2 filets to each plate. Pour ¼ cup coconut milk and sprinkle curry over each plate's filets. Chill 20 minutes and then serve.

Chicken Bruschetta

Prep time: 10 minutes

Cook time: 10 minutes

Serves: 4

INGREDIENTS

4 grass-fed chicken breasts

2 tomatoes

4 olives

2 onions

¼ tsp ground black pepper

1 cup roasted red pepper

3 tbsp extra virgin olive oil

INSTRUCTIONS

1. Dice the tomatoes, chop the olives and onions, and combine them
   with ground black pepper and 2 tbsp olive oil in a bowl and mix

well into a bruschetta. Puree the roasted red pepper in a blender and set aside.

2. Combine the chicken with 1 tbsp extra virgin olive oil and cook in a pan over medium-high heat for 4 minutes, turn once, and cook another 4-6 minutes, removing from heat while still tender.

3. Place one piece of chicken on each plate and pour the roasted red pepper over each, adding bruschetta over the top. Garnish with basil and serve.

Eggplant with Pesto Topping

Prep time: 10 minutes

Cook time: 8 minutes

Serves: 4

INGREDIENTS

1 large, thick eggplant

6-8 tomatoes

4 tbsp olive oil

¼ cup fresh basil

2 cloves garlic

INSTRUCTIONS

1. Preheat the grill. Slice the eggplant lengthwise into ½" thick slices, or ensuring that you have 4 slices. Slice the tomatoes into ¼" thick slices. Combine 4 tbsp olive oil with basil and garlic in a food processor and puree together.

2. Grill the eggplant until browned, turning once, about 3-4 minutes per side.

3. Remove eggplant from the grill and lay the tomato slices out over each piece. Top with the pesto puree and serve.

Salmon with Berry Chutney

Prep time: 10 minutes

Cook time: 15 minutes

Serves: 4

INGREDIENTS

4 salmon filets

16 stalks of asparagus

1 cup blueberries

1 onion

1 clove garlic

1 tbsp ginger root

¼ cup apple cider vinegar

½ tsp cinnamon

INSTRUCTIONS

1. Preheat your broiler. Finely chop the onion, garlic and ginger.
   Prepare a stove-top pot to steam the asparagus.

2. Combine blueberry, onion, garlic, ginger, apple cider vinegar and cinnamon in a saucepan and bring to a simmer, stirring continuously. Remove from heat once it has thickened into a sauce and set aside to cool.

3. Steam the asparagus for 3-5 minutes and broil the fish for 5-7 minutes. Remove from oven.

4. Lay one piece of fish across each plate and pour the blueberry chutney over top. Lay 4 stalks of asparagus over each piece of fish and serve.

Spicy Zucchini Eggplant Dine

Prep time: 15 minutes

Cook time: 20 minutes

Serves: 4

INGREDIENTS

3 small zucchini

1 eggplant

2 green peppers

6 tomatoes

1 onion

2 medium carrots

1 four-inch sweet orange pepper

1 cup water

1 tbsp extra virgin olive oil

INSTRUCTIONS

1. Using a julienne peeler, peel zucchini, eggplant and green peppers. Green peppers may be too tough for a julienne peeler, in which case try to simulate the effect of one using a knife. Combine the above in a pan with extra virgin olive oil and saute over medium heat, stirring, for 5 minutes.

2. Meanwhile, cut tomatoes into quarters, carrots into ½" thick slices, dice sweet pepper and dice onion. In a saucepan, combine the above with water and cook over medium heat until carrot is tender, about 15 minutes. Once finished, blend using an immersion blender, or pour into a blender and puree.

3. Pour the sauce over the zucchini, eggplant and peppers and serve.

Lettuce Nut Salad

Prep time: 10 min

Cook time: 6-8 minutes

Serves: 4

INGREDIENTS

1 7oz bag of Romaine lettuce

1 cup strawberries

1 cup blueberries

1 cup kiwi

½ cup almonds

½ cup walnuts

2 cups coconut milk

1 tbsp arrowroot

1 tsp cinnamon

¼ tsp chipotle chili pepper powder

INSTRUCTIONS

1. Dice the fruits. In a saucepan, combine coconut milk, arrowroot, cinnamon and chipotle chili pepper powder over medium heat. Cook, stirring, for 4 minutes. Add the walnuts and almonds to the sauce and continue cooking until slightly thick.

2. Combine lettuce and fruit in a bowl and drizzle the sauce over the top. Serve immediately or chill 20 minutes and then serve.

Baked Tilapia Filets

Prep time: 10 minutes

Cook time: 15 minutes

Serves: 4

INGREDIENTS

4 filets of tilapia

¼ tsp chipotle chili pepper powder

1 lemon

1 cup coconut milk

1 clove garlic

1 tsp lemon juice

2 tbsp dill

¼ tsp black ground pepper

INSTRUCTIONS

1. Preheat oven to 350 degrees. Chop the garlic and the dill and cut the lemon into slices.

2. Season tilapia with chipotle chili pepper powder and black ground pepper. Bake for 15 minutes or until tilapia flakes with a fork.

3. Combine coconut milk, garlic, lemon juice and dill in a bowl.

4. Remove fish from oven and pour sauce over the top, placing a lemon wedge over each. Serve immediately or chill 20 minutes and then serve.

Comfort Food Cookbook

Pancake Bacon Breakfast

Prep Time: 5 minutes

Cook Time: 25 minutes

Servings: 2

INGREDIENTS

8 slices nitrate-free bacon

Raw honey, agave nectar or date butter (optional)

Pancakes

1 1/4 cups almond flour

2 cage-free eggs

1/2 cup nut milk

2 tablespoons raw honey (or agave, date butter or stevia)

1 teaspoon baking powder

1 teaspoon vanilla

1/4 teaspoon Celtic sea salt

Coconut oil (for cooking)

Raw, agave or date butter (for garnish, optional)

INSTRUCTIONS

1. Heat large pan or skillet over medium-high heat.
2. Place bacon in hot pan and cook until crisp, about 4 - 5 minutes on each side. Remove bacon from pan and place on paper towel to drain. Reserve bacon fat in pan to cook *Pancakes*.

3. For *Pancakes*, in medium mixing bowl, beat eggs, nut milk, sweetener and vanilla with hand mixer or whisk. Add almond flour, salt and baking powder. Beat until smooth.

4. Use ladle or dry measure cup to pour batter onto hot oiled skillet. Fit 3 - 4 pancakes comfortably, so they do not touch as they spread.

5. Cook until edges are firm and batter bubbles slightly, about 3 - 4 minutes.

6. Carefully flip pancakes with spatula and cook for 1 - 2 minutes, or until cooked through. Repeat with remaining batter. Add coconut oil to pan, if necessary.

7. Transfer *Pancakes* and bacon to serving dish. Top with sweetener of choice and serve immediately.

Breakfast steak and Eggs

Prep Time: 5 minutes

Cook Time: 20 minutes

Servings: 1

INGREDIENTS

8 oz (1/2 lb) grass-fed bone-in steak (about 1 inch thick)

2 cage-free eggs

Celtic sea salt, to taste

Cracked black pepper, to taste

Coconut oil or bacon fat (for cooking)

INSTRUCTIONS

1. Heat cast iron pan or skillet over medium heat.
2. Sprinkle steak with salt and cracked black pepper on both sides. Place in hot pan and sear about 5 - 7 minutes per side for medium doneness. Flip steak halfway through cooking.
3. Remove steak from hot pan and allow to rest on cutting board or plate for a few minutes.
4. Heat medium pan over medium-high heat. Add 1 heaping tablespoon bacon fat or coconut oil to hot pan.
5. Gently add eggs to hot oiled pan and cover with well fitting lid. Decrease heat to medium-low and let eggs cook about 3 minutes for over-medium doneness.
6. Carefully release eggs from pan with spatula and transfer to serving dish. Top with cracked black pepper, to taste. Transfer rested steak to serving dish and serve hot.

Midnight Chicken and Waffles

Prep Time: 20 minutes

Cook Time: 15 minutes

Servings: 2

INGREDIENTS

Waffles

1 cup almond flour

1/4 coconut flour

3 cage-free eggs (separated)

1/4 cup coconut oil (or coconut or cacao butter, melted)

1/4 cup raw honey (or agave, date butter or stevia)

2 teaspoons aluminum-free baking soda

1 teaspoon vanilla

Pinch Celtic sea salt

Coconut oil (for cooking)

Raw honey, agave, fruit syrup (for garnish, optional)

Chicken Strips

8 oz (1/2 lb) boneless, skinless chicken (white or dark meat)

1 cage-free egg

1/2 cup coarse almond meal (or almond flour)

1 teaspoon flax meal

1/2 teaspoon paprika

1/2 teaspoon ground black pepper

1/2 teaspoon Celtic sea salt

1/4 teaspoon cayenne pepper (optional)

INSTRUCTIONS

1. Preheat waffle iron. Use wadded paper towel to carefully coat cooking surface with coconut oil. Heat medium pan over medium-high heat. Lightly coat pan with coconut oil.

2. For *Waffles*, in medium mixing bowl, beat egg whites to medium-stiff peaks with hand mixer, about 5 minutes.

3. In small mixing bowl, combine flours, salt and baking soda. In large mixing bowl, beat together egg yolks, oil or butter, sweetener and vanilla with hand mixer or whisk.

4. Beat flour mixture into egg yolk mixture. Gently fold egg whites into egg yolk batter.

5. Pour portion of batter onto hot waffle iron. Do not overfill. Cook 4 - 5 minutes, until golden brown and crisp. Repeat with remaining batter. Set aside cooked *Waffles*.

7. For *Chicken Strips*, cut chicken into equal portions. Add almond meal, flax meal, salt spices and to shallow dish and blend.

8. Add egg to separate shallow dish and beat. Dip and coat chicken in beaten egg, then dredge and coat well in almond meal mixture.

9. Carefully place coated chicken in hot oiled pan. Cook until golden brown and cooked through, about 3 - 4 minutes per side, depending on thickness. Turn with tongs halfway through cooking.

10. Remove *Chicken Strips* from pan and place on paper towel to drain.

11. Transfer cooked *Waffles* to serving dish. Top with *Chicken Strips*. Drizzle with raw honey, agave, or your favorite fruit syrup (optional).

12. Serve immediately.

Avocado Egg Salad

Prep Time: 5 minutes

Cook Time: 15 minutes

Servings: 4

INGREDIENTS

8 cage-free eggs

1 avocado

1 celery stalk

1/4 sweet onion

1/4 cup sweet pickle relish (or dill pickle relish + 1 tablespoon raw honey, agave or date butter)

1/4 cup organic mustard

2 teaspoons paprika

1/2 teaspoon ground black pepper

1/4 teaspoon Celtic sea salt

INSTRUCTIONS

1. Bring medium pot of lightly salted water to a boil. Leave enough room in pot for eggs.

2. Gently add eggs to hot water with tongs and cook about 10 minutes.

3. Drain eggs into colander in sink. Fill pot with cold water and add eggs back to pot. Let cold water run slowly over eggs in pot to cool.

4. Slice and pit avocado. Scoop flesh into medium mixing bowl. Thinly slice celery. Peel and finely dice onion. Add to mixing bowl

with relish, mustard, salt and spices. Mix with large spoon to combine.

5. Crack cooled eggs and peel off shells. Add boiled eggs to medium mixing bowl.

6. Use a fork or knife to chop eggs. Use large spoon to mix and mash ingredients together until smooth mixture with soft chunks forms. Stir to combine.

7. Transfer to serving dish and serve immediately. Or refrigerate about 20 minutes and serve chilled.

Grilled Cheese Sandwich

Prep Time: 20 minutes*

Cook Time: 60 minutes

Servings: 6

INGREDIENTS

White Bread

1 1/3 cups arrowroot powder

1 1/4 cups almond flour

4 cage-free eggs

4 cage-free egg whites

1/4 cup coconut oil (or cacao or coconut butter, melted)

2 teaspoons apple cider vinegar (or coconut vinegar or aminos)

1 1/2 tablespoons baking powder

1/2 tablespoon Celtic sea salt

Coconut oil (for cooking)

Cheese

1 1/2 cup cashews

1/4 cup nutritional yeast

1 lemon

1/2 teaspoon mustard powder

1/2 teaspoon ground white pepper (or ground black pepper)

1/2 teaspoon Celtic sea salt

Water

INSTRUCTIONS

1. *Soak cashews in enough water to cover for at least 4 hours, or overnight in refrigerator. Drain and rinse.
2. Preheat oven to 350 degrees F. Coat medium loaf pan with coconut oil.
3. For *White Bread*, in large mixing bowl, beat egg whites with whisk or hand mixer until frothy, about 1 minute. Add eggs, oil and vinegar and beat until light and thickened, about 2 minutes.
4. Sift arrowroot powder, almond flour, baking powder and salt into medium mixing bowl. Slowly stir flour mixture into egg mixture. Mix until well combined.
5. Pour batter into prepared loaf pan and bake for about 40 minutes, or until toothpick inserted into center comes out clean. Remove pan from oven and set aside to cool.
6. For *Cheese*, juice lemon into food processor or high-speed blender. Add cashews, nutritional yeast, salt and spices to processor. Process until smooth, about 2 minutes. Add enough water to reach thick, smooth consistency. Set aside.
7. Heat large pan over medium heat.
8. Once *White Bread* is cool slightly, insert knife around edges and remove from pan. Cut of ends of loaf, then cut into 12 slices.
9. Spread oil or butter on one side of each *White Bread* slice. Spread thick *Cheese* on bare side of each slice. Place slices together on cheese side.
10. Carefully place each sandwich in hot pan and grill until browned, about 2 - 3 minutes per side.
11. Transfer to serving dish and serve immediately.

Cheesy Southern Jalapeño "Cornbread"

Prep Time: 5 minutes

Cook Time: 25 minutes

Servings: 12

INGREDIENTS

1 1/2 cups almond flour

3 cage-free eggs

1/2 cup coconut oil (or coconut or cacao butter, melted) (or sub 1/4 cup with unsweetened applesauce)

1/4 cup nutritional yeast

2 fresh jalapeños (or 1/4 cup pickled jalapeño slices)

2 tablespoons organic apple cider vinegar

2 teaspoons baking powder

1/2 teaspoon paprika

1/2 teaspoon ground turmeric or mustard (optional)

1/2 teaspoon ground white pepper (or ground black pepper)

INSTRUCTIONS

1. Preheat oven to 350 degrees F. Lightly coat baking dish or cast-iron pan with coconut oil.

2. Beat eggs in medium mixing bowl with hand mixer or whisk until thick and slightly frothy. Add oil or butter, nutritional yeast and vinegar. Mix well.

3. Mix in almond meal, baking powder, and spices until combined.

4. Remove stems from fresh jalapenos. Slice and remove seeds. Stir in fresh or pickled jalapeño slices.

5. Pour batter into prepared baking dish or pan and bake 30 -35 minutes, until edges are golden brown and top is firm.

6. Remove from oven. Slice and serve warm. Or allow to cool to temperature and serve.

Chili Con Carne

Prep Time: 5 minutes

Cook Time: 40 minutes

Servings: 4

INGREDIENTS

16 oz (1 lb) lean grass-fed ground beef (or elk, bison, turkey or chicken)

15 oz (1 can) organic tomato sauce

29 oz (2 cans) organic diced tomatoes

1 cup water

1 cup cashews

1 small onion

1 bell pepper

2 cloves garlic

2 tablespoons chili powder

1 1/2 tablespoons smoked paprika (or paprika)

1 tablespoon ground cumin

1 teaspoon Mexican oregano (or dried oregano)

1 teaspoon ground black pepper

1/2 teaspoon cayenne pepper

1 teaspoon Celtic sea salt

1 tablespoon coconut oil

INSTRUCTIONS

1. Heat medium pot over medium-high heat. Add 1 tablespoon coconut oil to hot pan.

2. Peel onion and garlic. Remove stems, seeds and veins from bell pepper. Roughly chop and add to food processor or high-speed blender. Pulse until finely minced.

3. Add minced veggies to hot skillet and sauté for about 1 minute. Add ground beef and spices. Brown beef for about 5 minutes. Stir with whisk to break up meat well, or wooden spoon to keep beef chunkier.

4. Add whole cans of diced tomatoes and tomato sauce, and water. Stir to combine.

5. Bring to a simmer, then reduce heat to medium and cover pot loosely with lid to prevent splatter. Simmer about 30 minutes. Stir occasionally.

6. Remove from heat and transfer to serving dish. Use large serving spoon or ladle to serve hot.

Sweet Potato Cheese Fries

Prep Time: 10 minutes*

Cook Time: 35 minutes

Servings: 2

INGREDIENTS

Sweet Potato Fries

1 large sweet potato

2 tablespoons coconut oil

1/2 teaspoon smoked paprika

1/2 teaspoon ground black pepper

1/2 teaspoon Celtic sea salt

Coconut oil (for cooking)

Cheese Sauce

3/4 cup cashews

2 tablespoons nutritional yeast

1/2 lemon

1/4 teaspoon mustard powder

1/4 teaspoon cayenne pepper

1/4 teaspoon ground white pepper (or ground black pepper)

1/4 teaspoon Celtic sea salt

Water

INSTRUCTIONS

1. *Soak cashews in enough water to cover for at least 4 hours, or overnight in refrigerator. Drain and rinse.

2. Preheat oven to 450 degrees F. Line sheet pan with parchment or coat lightly with coconut oil.

3. For *Sweet Potato Fries*, peel sweet potato if preferred, but do not rinse. Slice sweet potato into 1/4 inch sticks and add to medium mixing bowl with coconut oil and spices. Toss to coat.

4. Spread potatoes in well-spaced, single layer on prepared sheet pan. Sprinkle salt evenly over potatoes and bake for 10 minutes.

5. Carefully remove sheet pan from oven and turn fries over with tongs or spatula. Back another 10 minutes, or until golden and crispy.

6. For *Cheese Sauce*, juice lemon into food processor or high-speed blender. Add cashews, nutritional yeast, salt and spices to processor. Process until smooth, about 2 minutes. Add enough water to reach desired consistency. Transfer to serving dish.

7. Remove *Sweet Potato Fries* from oven and transfer to serving dish. Serve immediately with *Cheese Sauce*.

Portobello Overload Burger

Prep Time: 10 minutes

Cook Time: 35 minutes

Servings: 2

INGREDIENTS

4 large Portobello mushroom caps

12 oz grass-fed ground beef (or chicken, turkey, bison, elk, etc.)

1/2 white onion

Cracked black pepper, to taste

Celtic sea salt, to taste

Coconut oil (for cooking)

Portobello Cheese Sauce

4 Portobello stems

3/4 cup cashews

2 tablespoons nutritional yeast

1/2 lemon

1/4 teaspoon mustard powder

1/4 teaspoon ground white pepper (or ground black pepper)

1/4 teaspoon Celtic sea salt

Water

Bacon fat or coconut oil (for cooking)

INSTRUCTIONS

1. *Soak cashews in enough water to cover for at least 4 hours, or overnight in refrigerator. Drain and rinse.

2. Preheat oven to 450 degrees F. Heat small pan over medium heat. Add 1 tablespoon bacon fat or coconut oil to hot pan. Line sheet pan with aluminum foil. Place metal cooling or baking rack over lined sheet pan.

3. Remove stems from Portobello mushroom caps. Chop and reserve stems. Place mushroom caps gill-side up on prepared sheet pan. Drizzle caps lightly with coconut oil.

4. Peel onion and slice crosswise into 2 full 1/4 inch cross sections. Keep rings intact and place on prepared sheet pan. Drizzle slightly with coconut oil and sprinkle with salt and pepper.

5. Form ground beef into 3/4 inch patties. Place on prepared sheet pan and sprinkle with salt and pepper.

6. Bake about 12 minutes, for medium-well burgers. Remove from oven and sprinkle mushroom caps with salt and pepper.

7. For *Portobello Cheese Sauce*, add chopped mushrooms stems to hot oiled pan. Sauté until soft and lightly caramelized, about 5 minutes. Stir occasionally.

8. Juice lemon into food processor or high-speed blender. Add cashews, nutritional yeast, salt and spices to processor. Process until smooth, about 2 minutes. Add enough water to reach desired consistency.

9. Add mixture to sautéed mushrooms and stir to heat *Portobello Cheese Sauce* through, about 2 minutes. Remove from heat.

10. Transfer 2 mushroom caps to serving dish, gill-side up. Top with roasted onion ring slice, then hamburger patty. Spoon *Portobello Cheese Sauce* over patty and top with remaining Portobello caps, gill-side down.

11. Serve hot.

Spicy Meatballs and Tomato Sauce

Prep Time: 5 minutes

Cook Time: 20 minutes

Servings: 4

INGREDIENTS

Meatballs

16 oz (1 lb) lean ground meat (beef, pork, chicken, turkey, bison, or any combination)

3/4 cup almond flour

1 cage-free egg

1/2 small onion (white, yellow or red)

1/2 teaspoon garlic powder

1/2 teaspoon cayenne pepper

1 teaspoon dried parsley

1 teaspoon dried oregano

1 teaspoon paprika

1 teaspoon red pepper flakes

1 teaspoon ground black pepper

1 teaspoon Celtic sea salt

1 tablespoon coconut oil

1 sprig fresh basil (for garnish, optional)

Tomato Sauce

14.5 oz (1 can) organic diced tomatoes

8 oz (1 can) organic tomato sauce

1 garlic clove

1/2 teaspoon dried oregano

1/2 teaspoon dried basil

1/2 teaspoon red pepper flakes

1/2 teaspoon ground black pepper

1 teaspoon coconut oil

INSTRUCTIONS

1. Heat large pan over medium heat. Add 1 tablespoon coconut oil to hot pan. Heat medium saucepan over medium heat. Add 1 teaspoon coconut oil.

2. For *Tomato Sauce*, peel garlic and mince. Add to medium saucepan and sauté until just golden, about 30 seconds. Add diced tomatoes, tomato sauce, salt and spices. Simmer about 5 - 10 minutes, stirring occasionally.

3. For *Meatballs*, peel onion process in food processor or high-speed blender, or finely grate.

4. Add to large mixing bowl. Add egg, ground meat, almond flour, spices and salt. Mix well with hands or large wooden spoon.

5. Form 24 meatballs with scoop or tablespoon, then roll in hands. Add meatballs to hot large pan and brown for 10 minutes. Turn with spatula or tongs to cook on all sides.

6. Add *Meatballs* to *Tomato Sauce* and simmer another 5 minutes.

7. Transfer *Meatballs* to serving dish. Top with simmering *Tomato Sauce*. Garnish with fresh basil (optional).

8. Serve hot.

Pan-Fried Eggplant Parm

Prep Time: 10 minutes

Cook Time: 20 minutes

Servings: 4

INGREDIENTS

Eggplant

1 eggplant

2 cage-free eggs

1 1/2 cups almond flour

1 tablespoon garlic powder

1 teaspoon dried oregano

1/2 teaspoon dried parsley

Celtic sea salt, to taste

Ground black pepper, to taste

1 small sprig fresh basil (for garnish)

Coconut oil (for cooking)

Pasta Sauce

14.5 oz (1 can) organic diced tomatoes

8 oz (1 can) organic tomato sauce

2 garlic cloves

1 tablespoon oregano (dried or fresh)

1 teaspoons paprika

1 teaspoon ground black pepper

1/2 teaspoon Celtic sea salt

1 teaspoon coconut oil

Almond Parmesan

1 cup almonds

2 tablespoons nutritional yeast

1 teaspoon garlic powder

1/2 teaspoon Celtic sea salt

INSTRUCTIONS

1. Heat medium saucepan over medium heat. Add 1 teaspoon coconut oil to hot pan. Heat large pan over medium-high heat. Coat hot pan well with coconut oil.

2. For *Pasta Sauce*, peel and mince garlic, then add to medium pan. Sauté until golden and aromatic, about 1 minute. Then add diced tomatoes, tomato sauce, salt and spices. Simmer until sauce reduces to desired consistency, about 5 - 10 minutes. Stir occasionally, then remove from heat and set aside.

3. For *Eggplant*, sift almond flour and spices into shallow dish. Add eggs to small shallow bowl and whisk.

4. Cut eggplant crosswise into 1/3 inch disks. Sprinkle with salt and pepper. Dredge eggplant in almond mixture until well coated. Shake off excess flour, then dip in egg. Return to almond flour mixture, then carefully place in large hot oiled pan. Repeat until pan is full, but not crowded.

5. Pan-fry eggplant until golden brown, about 2 minutes on each side. Flip halfway through cooking. Transfer breaded eggplant to paper towels to drain. Repeat with remaining eggplant.

6. For *Almond Parmesan*, add all ingredients to food processor or high-speed blender. Process until desired consistency is reached, coarsely or finely ground. Set aside.

7. Transfer breaded eggplant to serving dishes. To assemble, place layer of eggplant on serving dish. Spoon layer of *Pasta Sauce* over eggplant. Sprinkle on *Almond Parmesan*. Repeat with two more layers each of *Eggplant, Pasta Sauce* and *Almond Parmesan*.

8. Remove basil leaves from stem, stack together, roll up tightly, the thinly slice crosswise. Top dish with extra *Almond Parmesan* and chiffon of fresh basil.

9. Serve hot.

Cashew Ricotta Lasagna

Prep Time: 20 minutes

Cook Time: 40 minutes

Servings: 4

INGREDIENTS

1 large zucchini

Meat Filling

8 oz (1/2 lb) lean ground meat (beef, pork, turkey, chicken, etc.)

1/4 small onion (white, yellow or red)

1 teaspoon dried oregano

1/2 teaspoon garlic powder

1/2 teaspoon dried basil

1/2 teaspoon ground black pepper

1/2 teaspoon Celtic sea salt

Tomato Sauce

6 oz (1 can) organic tomato paste

8 oz (1 can) organic tomato sauce

2 teaspoons dried oregano

1 teaspoon garlic powder

1/2 teaspoon paprika

1/2 teaspoon ground black pepper

1/2 teaspoon Celtic sea salt

Spinach Ricotta

2 cup cashews

1 cup frozen chopped spinach (thawed)

1 teaspoon ground white pepper (or black pepper)

1/2 teaspoon garlic powder

1/2 teaspoon onion powder

1/2 teaspoon dried basil

1/2 teaspoon Celtic sea salt

Water

INSTRUCTIONS

1. *Soak cashews in enough water to cover for at least 4 hours, or overnight in refrigerator. Drain and rinse.

2. Preheat oven to 350 degrees F. Heat medium pan over medium-high heat.

3. For *Meat Filling*, peel onion and grate or mince. Add to hot pan with ground meat, salt and spices. Sauté until meat is browned, about 5 - 8 minutes. Remove from heat and set aside.

4. For *Spinach Ricotta*, add soaked cashews, salt and spices to food processor or high-speed blender. Process until smooth, about 2 minutes. Add chopped spinach and pulse to incorporate. Set aside.

5. For *Pasta Sauce*, add all ingredients to medium mixing bowl and mix until combined. Set aside.

6. Slice zucchini lengthwise into 1/4 inch slices with mandolin or knife.

7. To assemble, layer a few spoonfuls of *Tomato Sauce* along bottom of baking dish. Top with layer of zucchini, *Spinach Ricotta, Meat Filling* and *Sauce*. Repeat process with remaining components.

End with a layer of zucchini, then *Sauce* on top. Add a dash of extra spices, if preferred.

8. Place *Lasagna* in oven and bake for about 40 minutes, until heated through. Remove from oven and let cool about 10 minutes.

9. Serve warm.

Italian Sausage and Peppers

Prep Time: 5 minutes

Cook Time: 20 minutes

Servings: 4

INGREDIENTS

4 large spicy Italian sausage links (pork, chicken or turkey)

1 yellow onion

1 green bell pepper

Cracked black pepper, to taste

INSTRUCTIONS

1. Heat large cast iron pan or skillet over medium heat.
2. Add sausage links to hot pan and sear on one side about 8 - 10 minutes.
3. Peel onion. Remove stems, seeds and veins from bell pepper. Chop or slice onion and pepper and add to pan.
4. Turn over sausage links and stir veggies. Sear sausage and sauté veggies until sausage is cooked through and veggies are tender and caramelized, about 8 - 10 minutes. Stir veggies around sausage occasionally. Try not to disturb sausage too much.
5. Transfer sausage to cutting board and slice into 1 1/2 inch pieces, if desired.
6. Transfer *Sausage and Peppers* to serving dish and serve hot.

Cashew Mac and "Cheese"

Prep Time: 15 minutes

Cook Time: 30 minutes

Servings: 4

INGREDIENTS

2 spaghetti squash (or summer squash or zucchini)

Cheese Sauce

1 1/2 cup cashews

1/4 cup nutritional yeast

1 lemon

1/4 teaspoon cayenne pepper

1/2 teaspoon mustard powder

1/2 teaspoon ground white pepper (or ground black pepper)

1/2 teaspoon Celtic sea salt

Water

Topping

1 cup almonds

2 tablespoons nutritional yeast

1/2 teaspoon mustard powder

1/2 teaspoon Celtic sea salt

Pinch cayenne pepper

INSTRUCTIONS

1. *Soak cashews in enough water to cover for at least 4 hours, or overnight in refrigerator. Drain and rinse.

2. Preheat oven to 350 degrees F. Bring large pot of salted water to boil over high heat.

3. Gently place squash into boiling water and cook until tender, about 15 minutes. Remove and submerge in cool water to cool. Set aside.

4. For *Cheese Sauce*, juice lemon into food processor or high-speed blender. Add cashews, nutritional yeast, salt and spices to processor. Process until smooth, about 2 minutes. Add enough water to reach desired consistency. Transfer to medium mixing bowl.

5. For *Topping*, add all ingredients to clean food processor or high-speed blender. Process to reach desired consistency. Mixture should be coarsely or finely ground. Set aside.

6. Remove seeds from cooled spaghetti squash, and use fork to shred. Or grate, julienne (thinly slice) or spiralize summer squash or zucchini. Add squash *Cheese Sauce* in mixing bowl. Gently mix to combine.

7. Transfer mixture to baking dish. Sprinkle *Topping* over dish.

8. Place in oven and bake for about 10 - 15 minutes, until heated through.

9. Remove from oven and serve warm.

Delicious Chicken Pot Pie

Prep Time: 25 minutes*

Cook Time: 45 minutes

Servings: 4

INGREDIENTS

Filling

16oz (1lb) boneless skin-on chicken (or pheasant, game hen, etc.)

2 cups chicken broth

2 large carrots

1 large celery stalk

1 green bell pepper

1 small onion

2 garlic cloves

1/2 lemon

1 cage-free egg

2 tablespoons tapioca flour

2 tablespoons coconut flour

2 teaspoons dried thyme (or 4 teaspoons fresh thyme)

1/2 teaspoon black pepper

Celtic sea salt (to taste)

Bacon fat or coconut oil (for cooking)

Crust

1 1/2 cup almond flour

1/2 cup coconut flour

3/4 cup cold coconut oil (or room temperature cacao butter)

3 cage-free eggs

2 teaspoons dried thyme

1 teaspoon Celtic sea salt

Water

INSTRUCTIONS

1. *For *Crust*, add almond and coconut flour, thyme and salt to medium mixing bowl. Cut oil or butter into flour with fork until crumbly. Mix in eggs until dough starts to combine together. Mix in enough water to bring together tender dough.

2. *Divide dough in half and roll into round disks. Place one dough round over pie pan or plate and gentle press in. Cover and place in freezer 1 hour. Cover and refrigerate remaining dough.

3. Preheat oven to 350 degrees F. Heat large pot over medium heat.

4. For *Filling*, add 2 tablespoons bacon fat or coconut oil to hot pot. Add chicken pieces skin-side down. Cook chicken until browned and fat renders out, about 5 minutes. Turn chicken over and continue cooking another 5 minutes. Remove chicken from pot and set aside.

5. Add coconut and tapioca flour to pot and whisk until smooth paste forms. Gradually whisk in chicken broth. Simmer about 5 minutes, whisking occasionally.

6. Peel and mince garlic. Peel onion and dice. Remove stems, seeds and veins from bell pepper, then chop. Dice carrots and celery. Add veggies to pot with thyme, salt, pepper and lemon juice.

7. Remove skin from par-cooked chicken and chop. Add back to pot.

8. Beat egg in small mixing bowl and slowly spoon in hot chicken stock to temper. Once egg is tempered, add to pot and stir to

incorporate. Simmer for 10 minutes, then remove from heat and set aside.

9. Remove *Crust* from freezer and refrigerator. Carefully ladle *Filling* into bottom frozen *Crust*. Lay top *Crust* over *Filling*. Pinch together and crimp edges of top and bottom *Crust* to seal.

10. Brush top *Crust* with bacon fat or coconut oil and sprinkle with salt. Use knife to cut a few slits in top *Crust*.

11. Bake for 35 - 45 minutes, or until crust is golden. Remove from oven and let to cool at least 15 minutes.

12. Serve warm.

Little Lamb Sheppard's Pie

Prep Time: 20 minutes

Cook Time: 60 minutes

Servings: 4

INGREDIENTS

Meat Filling

24 oz (1 1/2 lbs) grass-fed ground lamb (or beef, bison, elk, etc.)

1 cup chicken broth or stock (or beef brother or stock, or red wine)

1 large onion (yellow or white)

2 carrots

6 - 10 asparagus stalks (about 1/2 cup chopped)

1/2 sweet potato (about 1/2 cup diced)

2 garlic cloves

1 tablespoon organic tomato paste

1 teaspoon tamari (or coconut aminos)

2 tablespoons tapioca flour (or arrow root powder)

1 sprig fresh rosemary

1 sprig fresh thyme

1/2 teaspoon ground black pepper (or ground white pepper)

1 teaspoon Celtic sea salt

Bacon fat or coconut oil (for cooking)

Parsnip Topping

4 medium parsnips

1/2 medium onion (yellow or white)

2 tablespoons cacao butter (or coconut oil)

2 cups water

3/4 teaspoon Celtic sea salt

1/2 ground white pepper (or ground black pepper) (optional)

INSTRUCTIONS

1. Heat medium pot over medium heat. Add 2 tablespoons bacon fat or coconut oil to hot pot.

2. For *Meat Filling*, peel and mince garlic. Peel and chop onion. Dice carrots and sweet potato. Chop asparagus. Add to hot oiled pot and sauté about 5 minutes.

3. Add lamb, salt and spices to veggies. Brown lamb and sauté another 5 minutes. Whisk in tapioca flour and cook another minute.

4. Remove rosemary and thymes leaves from stems and add to pot with stock, tomato paste and tamari. Let simmer and thicken about 12 minutes.

5. Preheat oven to 400 degrees F. Heat large pan with lid over medium heat. Add butter or oil to hot pan.

6. For *Parsnip Topping*, peel and mince or finely grate onion. Add to hot pan and sauté until translucent and aromatic, about 2 minutes.

7. Peel and slice or chop parsnips. Add to onions with water. Increase heat to high and bring to a simmer. Cover pan loosely with lid. Cook parsnips partially covered until softened and most of the water has evaporated, about 10 minutes.

8. Pour parsnips and onions into food processor or high-speed blender. Process until thick, smooth mixture forms. Add enough water to reach desired consistency. Set aside.

9. Transfer *Meat Filling* to baking or casserole dish. Top with *Parsnip Topping*. Smooth over or create design with offset spatula or back of spoon.

10. Bake about 25 minutes, until *Parsnip Topping* is golden.

11. Remove from oven and let cool at least 10 minutes. Serve warm.

Country Chicken and Dumplings

Prep Time: 10 minutes

Cook Time: 40 minutes

Servings: 4

INGREDIENTS

Chicken Soup

16 oz (1 lb) skin-on bone-in chicken pieces

3 cups organic chicken broth or stock

3 cups water

2 carrots

2 celery stalks

1/2 small white onion

2 bay leaves

2 teaspoons dried thyme (or 4 teaspoons fresh thyme)

1/2 teaspoon paprika

1 teaspoon black pepper

1 teaspoon Celtic sea salt

Dumplings

1 1/2 cups almond flour

1/4 cup arrowroot powder

1 cage-free egg

1/4 cup chilled coconut oil (or room temperature coconut or cacao butter)

1/2 teaspoon baking soda

1/2 ground bay leaf

1/2 teaspoon garlic powder

1/2 teaspoon ground white pepper (or ground black pepper)

1/2 teaspoon Celtic sea salt

Nut milk or chicken broth or stock

INSTRUCTIONS

1. Heat large pot over medium-high heat. Place chicken skin-side down in hot pot. Sear and render out fat for about 5 minutes.

2. Chop carrots and celery. Peel onion and mince. Add veggies to chicken with salt and pepper.

3. Turn chicken over and brown on flesh side about 5 minutes. Stir veggies occasionally.

4. Add bay, thyme and paprika, chicken stock and water to pot. Increase heat to high and bring to a boil. Reduce heat and simmer about 25 minutes. Place lid loosely over pot to prevent splatter, if necessary.

5. For *Dumplings*, sift almond flour and arrowroot into medium mixing bowl. Cut in solid oil or butter with fork until crumbly mixture forms. Add egg, salt and spices, baking soda, and enough nut milk or chicken broth to bring together soft, slightly sticky dough.

6. Use tablespoon or small scoop to gently drop dough into *Chicken Soup*. Cover with well fitting lid and let simmer about 10 minutes.

7. Gently stir soup to prevent *Dumplings* from sticking. Turn over any *Dumplings* that are not submerged. Continue simmering 5 minutes, or until *Dumplings* are cooked through.

8. Remove from heat and transfer to serving dish. Use large serving spoon or ladle to serve hot.

All Day Country Fried Steak

Prep Time: 10 minutes

Cook Time: 15 minutes

Servings: 2

INGREDIENTS

Country Fried Steak

12 oz (3/4 lb) grass-fed beef (cube steak or fillet)

1 cage-free egg

1 teaspoon coconut aminos (or tamari)

1/3 cup arrowroot powder

1/4 cup macadamia nuts

1/4 cup pistachios (or almonds or cashews)

1/4 teaspoon garlic powder

1/4 teaspoon onion powder

1/4 teaspoon paprika

1/4 teaspoon cracked black pepper (or ground black pepper)

1/4 teaspoon Celtic sea salt

Pinch cayenne pepper

Pinch dried oregano

Coconut oil (for cooking)

Bacon fat (for cooking)

White Gravy

2 teaspoons arrowroot powder

5 oz (1/2 can) full-fat coconut milk

1/2 teaspoon Celtic salt

1/2 teaspoon ground white pepper (or ground black pepper)

Bacon fat

INSTRUCTIONS

1. Heat cast iron pan or skillet over medium-high heat. Add 1 tablespoon each bacon fat and coconut oil to hot pan.

2. For *Country Fried Steak*, add nuts to food processor or high-speed blender. Process until finely ground. Add arrowroot, salt and spices. Pulse to incorporated. Transfer mixture to shallow dish. Set aside.

3. In separate shallow dish, beat egg and coconut aminos. Set aside.

4. Tenderize beef fillet with tenderizing mallet, if using. Dip and coat cube steak in egg mixture, then dredge and coat well in nut mixture.

5. Place coated cube steak into hot oiled pan. Cook until golden and crisp, about 2 minutes on each side. Repeat with remaining steak. Remove cooked steak from pan and place on paper towel to drain.

6. For *White Gravy*, add enough bacon fat to hot skillet so there is about 2 - 3 tablespoons in pan. Allow to heat thoroughly.

7. Add arrowroot to pan. Whisk and cook for 1 minute. Whisk in coconut milk. Whisk and cook another minute. Whisk in salt and pepper. Remove from heat.

8. Transfer *Country Fried Steak* to serving dish. Top with *White Gravy* and serve hot.

Bacon Sautéed Liver and Onions

Prep Time: 20 minutes*

Cook Time: 25 minutes

Servings: 4

INSTRUCTIONS

20 oz (1 1/4 lb) calves liver

2 onions (yellow or white)

4 slices nitrate-free bacon

1 lemon

2 tablespoons arrowroot powder

1/2 teaspoon Celtic sea salt

1/2 teaspoon cracked black pepper (or ground black pepper)

Bacon fat or coconut oil (for cooking)

INSTRUCTIONS

1. *Remove thin outer membrane from liver and slice into 1/4 inch fillets. Add to glass container. Juice lemon into container and toss to coat. Cover well and refrigerate overnight.
2. Heat large cast-iron pan or skillet set over medium heat.
3. Cut bacon lengthwise into long, thin strips. Then cut in thirds crosswise and add to hot pan. Sauté bacon and let crisp, about 5 minutes. Stir occasionally. Decrease heat to medium-low.
4. Peel and thinly slice onions. Add to bacon and sauté until caramelized, about 10 minutes. Stir occasionally. Remove caramelized onions and bacon from pan and set aside.

5. Drain liver fillets in colander in sink. Rinse under running water, then pat dry.

6. In shallow dish, add arrowroot powder, salt and pepper. Mix with fork to combine.

7. Dredge liver slices in arrowroot mixture and shake off excess. Place coated liver fillets on a plate and coat remaining liver fillets.

8. Add 2 tablespoons bacon fat or coconut oil to hot pan. Add single layer of coated liver to hot oiled pan and sear for 1 minute per side. Place liver on paper towel to drain. Repeat with remaining liver.

9. Transfer liver to serving dish. Top with caramelized onions and bacon. Serve immediately .

Oven-Crunch Chicken

Prep Time: 10 minutes

Cook Time: 60 minutes

Servings: 4

INGREDIENTS

32 oz (2 lb) bone-in, skinless chicken

3/4 cup fine almond flour

3/4 cup coarse almond meal (or almond flour)

2 cage free eggs

1/3 cup nut milk

1/2 teaspoon cayenne pepper

1 teaspoon ground black pepper

1 1/2 teaspoons paprika

1 1/2 tablespoons Celtic sea salt

Coconut oil (in spray bottle)

INSTRUCTIONS

1. Preheat oven to 350 degrees F. Fill spray bottle with warm coconut oil.
2. Line sheet pan with aluminum foil. Place metal cooling or baking rack over lined sheet pan. Generously spray metal rack with coconut oil to coat. Set second sheet pan aside.
3. Add almond meal and/or flour to small mixing bowl with 1 tablespoon salt and spices. Mix to combine with fork or whisk to break up clumps.
4. In shallow dish, beat eggs and nut milk until combined.

5. Use serving spoon or measuring cup to dust second sheet pan with layer of almond flour mixture onto. Sprinkle chicken with 1/2 tablespoon salt.

6. Dip and coat all chicken pieces in egg mixture then lay on second sheet pan, over layer of almond flour mixture. Use spoon or measuring cut to sprinkle almond flour mixture from mixing bowl over dipped chicken. Pat almond flour mixture into chicken on all sides until well coated.

7. Transfer coasted chicken to prepared wire rack. Generously spray coated chicken with coconut oil.

8. Bake 60 - 70 minutes, until coating is crisp and chicken is cooked through. Remove from oven and allow to cool at least 10 minutes. Then place crispy chicken on paper towels to drain, if desired.

9. Transfer to serving dish and serve immediately.

Garlicky Mashed Parsnips

Prep Time: 10 minutes

Cook Time: 20 minutes

Servings: 4

INSTRUCTIONS

4 medium parsnips

1/2 white onion

4 garlic cloves

Celtic sea salt (to taste)

Ground black pepper (to taste)

Water

Bacon fat or coconut oil (for cooking)

INSTRUCTIONS

1. Heat large pan with lid over medium heat. Add 2 tablespoons bacon fat or coconut oil to hot pan.
2. Peel and mince or finely grate onion and garlic. Add to hot oiled pan and sauté until golden and aromatic, about 2 minutes.
3. Peel and slice or chop parsnips. Add to pan with 2 cups water. Increase heat to high and bring to a simmer. Cover pan loosely with lid. Cook partially covered until parsnips soften and most of the water has evaporated, about 10 minutes.
4. Pour parsnips, onions and garlic into food processor or high-speed blender. Process until thick, smooth mixture forms.
5. Transfer to serving dish and serve immediately.

Oven-Crisp Croquettes

Prep Time: 25 minutes*

Cook Time: 60 minutes

Servings: 8

INGREDIENTS

White Bread

1 1/3 cups arrowroot powder

1 1/4 cups almond flour

4 cage-free eggs

4 cage-free egg whites

1/4 cup coconut oil (or cacao or coconut butter, melted)

2 teaspoons apple cider vinegar (or coconut vinegar or aminos)

1 1/2 tablespoons baking powder

1/2 tablespoon Celtic sea salt

Chilled coconut oil (or room temperature coconut or cacao butter, for cooking)

Cheesy Filling

1/2 cup chopped cooked ham (or chicken, turkey, etc.)

4 slices nitrate-free bacon

1/2 onion (white, yellow or red)

3/4 cup cashews

1/4 cup nutritional yeast

1 lemon

1/2 teaspoon mustard powder

1/2 teaspoon cayenne pepper

1/2 teaspoon ground white pepper (or ground black pepper)

1/2 teaspoon Celtic sea salt

Water

INSTRUCTIONS

1. *Soak cashews in enough water to cover for at least 4 hours, or overnight in refrigerator. Drain and rinse.

2. Preheat oven to 350 degrees F. Coat baking dish with coconut oil.

3. For *White Bread*, in large mixing bowl, beat egg whites with whisk or hand mixer until frothy, about 1 minute. Add eggs, oil and vinegar and beat until light and thickened, about 2 minutes.

4. Sift arrowroot powder, almond flour, baking powder and salt into medium mixing bowl. Slowly stir flour mixture into egg mixture. Mix until well combined.

5. Pour batter into prepared baking pan and bake for about 30 minutes, or until toothpick inserted into center comes out clean. Remove pan from oven and set aside to cool.

6. Heat medium pan over medium-high heat. Line sheet pan with aluminum foil. Place metal cooling or baking rack over lined sheet pan. Generously spray metal rack with coconut oil to coat.

7. For *Cheesy Filling*, chop bacon and add to hot pan. Sauté until crisp and fat is rendered out, about 8 minutes. Transfer bacon to medium mixing bowl. Reserve bacon fat in pan.

8. Peel and mince or finely grate onion. Add to hot oiled pan and sauté until translucent and aromatic, about 5 minutes.

9. Add chopped, cooked meat to pan and sauté until warm, about 2 minutes. Remove from heat and add to mixing bowl.

10. Juice lemon into food processor or high-speed blender. Add cashews, nutritional yeast, salt and spices to processor. Process until smooth, about 2 minutes. Add enough water to reach desired consistency. Add to mixing bowl.

11. Remove *White Bread* from baking dish. Cut in half. Dice one portion. Add to *Cheesy Filling* and mix to combine. Mixture should be moist and stick together when pressed. Add nut milk or water to reach desired consistency, if necessary.

12. Form mixture into golf ball-sized rounds and place on plate.

13. Chop remaining *White Bread* and add to clean food processor high-speed blender. Pulse to coarsely grind and add to empty mixing bowl. Roll *Cheesy Filling* balls in ground *White Bread*. Pat to secure coating and transfer to prepared wire rack. Spray *Croquettes* with coconut oil.

14. Bake about 20 minutes, until outside is golden brown and crisp. Remove from oven and transfer to serving dish.

15. Serve hot.

Tropical Beef Patty

Prep Time: 25 minutes

Cook Time: 30 minutes

Servings: 4

INSTRUCTIONS

Crust

2 cups almond flour

2 cage-free eggs

3 tablespoons chilled coconut oil (or room temperature coconut or cacao butter)

1 teaspoon turmeric

1/4 teaspoon baking soda

1/2 teaspoon Celtic sea salt

Filling

12 oz (3/4 lb) grass-fed beef (ground or fillet)

1/2 small onion (yellow, white or red)

1 tablespoon tamari (or coconut aminos)

1 tablespoon raw honey (or agave or date butter)

1 tablespoon curry powder

1 teaspoon allspice

1 teaspoon chili powder

1 teaspoon red pepper flake

1/2 teaspoon garlic powder

1/2 teaspoon onion powder

1/2 teaspoon Celtic sea salt

INSTRUCTIONS

1. For *Crust*, sift almond flour into medium mixing bowl. Add baking soda, turmeric and salt.

2. Whisk eggs in small mixing bowl, then add to flour and combine. Slowly cut in coconut oil with fork until malleable dough comes together.

3. Roll dough in plastic wrap or wrap tightly in parchment and refrigerate for 15 minutes.

4. Preheat oven to 400 degrees F. Line sheet pan with parchment or baking mat. Cover cutting board with parchment. Heat medium pan over medium heat.

5. For *Filling*, grind or mince beef fillet, if using. Peel and mince or finely grate onion. Add onion and beef to hot pan with salt and spices. Sauté until beef is browned and onions are soft, about 8 minutes. Use whisk to break up meat well, or wooden spoon to keep chunkier form. Remove from heat and set aside.

6. Remove dough from refrigerator and divide into 4 portions. Roll dough into balls and use hands to flatten on prepared cutting board. Roll into circles about 1/8 inch thick with rolling pin.

7. Scoop equal portions of *Filling* into center of one half of dough circle. Fold bare half of dough over filled half. Press edges together, letting any trapped air escape. Crimp edges of dough together with fork. Repeat with remaining dough.

8. Arrange patties on lined sheet pan and bake 15 - 20 minutes, until dough is golden and cooked through. Remove from oven transfer to serving dish.

9. Serve hot.

Sweet Banana Bread

Prep Time: 5 minutes

Cook Time: 40 minutes

Servings: 8

INGREDIENTS

1 cup almond flour

1/4 cup coconut flour

2 overripe bananas

2 cage-free eggs

1/4 cup raw honey (or agave, date butter or stevia)

1/4 cup coconut oil (or coconut or cacao butter, melted) (or unsweetened applesauce or nut butter)

1 tablespoon baking powder

2 teaspoons ground cinnamon

1/2 teaspoon ground nutmeg

1 teaspoon vanilla

1/2 teaspoon Celtic sea salt

INSTRUCTIONS

1. Preheat oven to 350 degrees F. Coat small or medium loaf pan with coconut oil.

2. Peel bananas and add to medium mixing bowl. Beat with hand mixer or whisk. Add eggs, oil or butter, and sweetener. Beat well, about 1 - 2 minutes.

3. In separate bowl, blend flours, baking powder, salt and spices. Pour banana mixture into flour mixture and stir to combine.

4. Pour batter into prepared loaf pan and bake for 30 - 40 minutes, or until browned and firm in the center.

5. Remove from oven and set aside to cool.

6. Slice and serve warm. Or allow to cool completely and serve room temperature.

Pumpkin Spice Bread

Prep Time: 5 minutes

Cook Time: 40 minutes

Servings: 8

INGREDIENTS

1 cup almond flour

3/4 cup coconut flour

15 oz (1 can) pumpkin puree

2 cage-free eggs

1/2 cup nut milk

1/2 cup unsweetened applesauce

1/4 cup coconut oil (or coconut or cacao butter, melted) (or nut butter)

1/4 cup raw honey (or agave, date butter or stevia)

1/4 cup pumpkin seeds

2 teaspoons baking soda

1 tablespoon ground cinnamon

1 teaspoon ground nutmeg

1 teaspoon Celtic sea salt

1/2 teaspoon ground black pepper (optional)

Coconut oil (for cooking)

INSTRUCTIONS

1. Preheat oven to 350 degrees F. Coat medium loaf pan with coconut oil.

2. Add eggs, oil or butter, applesauce, nut milk and sweetener to food processor or high-speed blender. Process until thick and light, about 1 - 2 minutes.
3. Add pumpkin, salt and spices. Process to incorporate.
4. Add flour and baking soda to small mixing bowl and stir to combine. Add to processor in batches and process until well combined.
5. Pour batter into prepared loaf pan and bake 35 - 40 minutes, until firm but springy in the center.
6. Remove from oven and set aside to cool.
7. Slice and serve warm. Or allow to cool completely and serve room temperature.

Asian Cookbook

Cashew Chicken Satay

Prep Time: 10 minutes*

Cook Time: 25 minutes

Servings: 4

INGREDIENTS

16 oz (1 lb) boneless skinless chicken

12 wooden skewers (soaked in water for 1 hour)

Marinade

1 tablespoon pure fish sauce (or liquid aminos or coconut Aminos)

2 inch piece fresh ginger rot

1 garlic clove

Satay Sauce

13 oz (1 can) full-fat coconut milk

1/2 cup crunchy almond butter

1 tablespoon raw honey or agave nectar

1 tablespoon pure fish sauce (or tamari or coconut aminos)

1 teaspoon apple cider vinegar (or liquid aminos or coconut vinegar)

4 shallots

2 garlic cloves

2 inch piece fresh ginger root

2 small red chili peppers

1 1/2 tablespoons lime juice

Coconut oil (for cooking)

INSTRUCTIONS

1. *Cut chicken into 1 inch strips. For *Marinade*, peel and mince garlic and ginger. Add to medium mixing bowl with fish sauce and whisk. Add chicken and toss with until coated. Cover and set aside to marinate for 1 hour.

2. *Soak wooden skewers in water in shallow dish for 1 hour.

3. Heat medium pan or wok over medium heat and add 1 tablespoon coconut oil.

4. For *Satay Sauce*, peel and mince shallots, garlic and ginger. Slice peppers. Add to hot pan and sauté until softened, about 5 - 8 minutes.

5. Reduce heat to low. Add almond butter, coconut milk, honey, fish sauce, vinegar and lime juice. Whisk until blended. Gently simmer for 10 minutes. Remove from heat, but keep warm.

6. Preheat outdoor grill or griddle pan over medium-high heat. Lightly coat with coconut oil.

7. Pierce marinated chicken strips with soaked skewers. Pour some *Satay Sauce* over chicken and brush lightly with marinade brush to coat. Transfer remaining *Satay Sauce* to serving dish.

8. Grill chicken on preheated grill until just cooked through, about 3 minutes per side. Turn over skewers halfway through cooking. Do not overcook.

9. Remove skewers from heat and transfer to serving dish. Serve with *Satay Sauce*.

Savory BBQ Pork Bun

Prep Time: 15 minutes

Cook Time: 90 minutes

Servings: 8

INGREDIENTS

Buns

2 cups tapioca flour (plus extra)

1/2 cup coconut flour (plus extra)

2 cage-free eggs

1 cup warm water

1/2 cup coconut oil

1/2 cup unsweetened applesauce

2 teaspoons apple cider vinegar

1 teaspoon baking soda

1 teaspoon Celtic sea salt

Filling

16 oz (1 lb) bone-in pork (shoulder, ribs, rump, etc.)

14 oz (1 can) organic crushed tomatoes

8 oz (1 can) organic tomato sauce

2 apples

1/2 large onion (white or yellow)

2 tablespoons raw honey (agave or date butter)

1 tablespoon apple cider vinegar (or tamari or coconut aminos)

1 garlic clove

3 tablespoons paprika

1 teaspoon ground black pepper

2 teaspoons Celtic sea salt

Coconut oil (for cooking)

INSTRUCTIONS

1. Heat medium pot over medium-high heat. Add 1 tablespoon coconut oil to hot pan.

2. For *Filling*, add bone-in pork to pot and sear on all sides, about 10 minutes.

3. Peel, core and dice apples. Peel onion and garlic. Add to food processor or high-speed blender with crushed tomatoes. Process until smooth, about 1 - 2 minutes.

4. Pour tomato mixture into pot. Add tomato sauce, honey, vinegar, salt and spices. Stir and bring to a simmer.

5. Reduce heat to low and cover loosely with lid. Simmer for about 1 hour, until meat is tender and liquid is reduced and thickened. Stir occasionally.

6. Remove pot from heat. Remove pork from sauce, cut off bone, and shred or chop. Add meat back to pot and stir to combine. Set aside.

7. Preheat oven to 350 degrees F. Line sheet pan with parchment paper or coat with coconut oil.

8. For *Buns*, sift together tapioca flour, coconut flour, baking soda and salt in medium bowl. Stir in warm water and oil.

9. Whisk eggs and vinegar in small bowl. Add egg mixture to flour mixture and mix to form soft, slightly sticky dough. Add water or coconut flour 1 tablespoon at a time to reach desired consistency, if necessary.

10. Divide dough into 8 portions and flatten into round disks. Dust hands or rolling pin with extra tapioca flour to prevent sticking.

11. Use tongs to place *Filling* into center of dough. Bring up edges of dough around *Filling* and pinch together to create round, sealed ball.

12. Place filled *Buns* sealed-side down on sheet pan and pat down slightly. Bake 20 minutes, until edges are golden brown and dough is cooked through.

13. Remove from oven and serve hot. Or let cool slightly and serve warm.

Easy Kimchi

Prep Time: 30 minutes*

Servings: 8

INGREDIENTS

1 (2 lb) cabbage head (napa or other variety)

1/2 cup Celtic sea salt

Water

Pepper Sauce

1/3 cup red pepper flakes

1/4 cup pure fish sauce

8 garlic cloves

3 green onions (scallions)

1/2 carrot

1 tablespoon raw honey (or agave)

INSTRUCTIONS

1. Chop cabbage into thin strips and add to large mixing bowl.
2. Add 1 cup cold water and salt to bowl. Mix well with hands. Set aside for 10 minutes.
3. For *Pepper Sauce*, peel and mince garlic. Chop green onions. Julienne (thinly slice lengthwise) carrot. Add to lidded container with pepper, fish sauce, and honey. Mix to combine.
4. Drain cabbage in colander. Rinse in cold water several times. Add cabbage to *Pepper Sauce* and toss well to coat.
5. Transfer to serving dish and serve immediately.

6. *Or press down into container with hands and cover with air-tight lid. Set aside at room temperature to ferment for several days. Then serve.

Japanese Seaweed Salad

Prep Time: 10 minutes

Servings: 2

INGREDIENTS

1 oz dry mixed seaweed

1 1/2 tablespoons coconut vinegar (or apple cider vinegar)

1 tablespoon tamari (or coconut aminos or liquid aminos)

1/2 tablespoon raw honey (or agave)

1 tablespoon sesame oil

1/2 piece fresh ginger (1/2 teaspoon ginger juice)

1 green onion (scallion)

1 tablespoon sesame seeds (toasted, if preferred)

Celtic sea salt, to taste

Water

INSTRUCTIONS

1. Add seaweed to large mixing bowl with at least 2 cups cold water. Set aside 5 minutes for crunchy texture, or 10 minutes for softer texture.

2. Juice fresh ginger. Add vinegar, tamari, honey, sesame oil, ginger juice and salt to small mixing bowl. Whisk to combine. Set aside.

3. Heat small pan over medium heat. Add sesame seeds to hot dry pan. Toast about 2 minutes, stirring frequently. Remove from heat and transfer to small dish. Set aside.

4. Drain seaweed in colander or strainer and squeeze out excess water with hands. Use paper towel to remove any extra water from bowl.

Return hydrated seaweed to bowl with tamari mixture and sesame seeds. Toss well to combine. Transfer to serving dish.

5. Thinly slice scallions and sprinkle over dish. Serve immediately.

Asian Meatball Snacks

Prep Time: 10 minutes

Cook Time: 20 minutes

Servings: 4

INGREDIENTS

32 oz (2 lbs) ground meat (beef, pork, chicken, bison, or any combination)

1/2 cup almond flour

2 eggs

2 teaspoons sesame oil (or coconut or almond oil)

2 garlic cloves

4 large green onions (scallions)

1 teaspoon sesame seeds

1/2 teaspoon ground ginger

Sauce

2/3 cup pure fish sauce (or tamari)

1/4 cup coconut vinegar (or apple cider vinegar)

2 tablespoons raw honey (or agave)

2 garlic cloves

1 teaspoon sesame oil

1 teaspoon ground ginger

DIRECTIONS

1. Preheat oven to 400 degrees F. Line baking sheet with parchment or baking mat.

2. Peel garlic and cut 1 green onion in half. Thinly slice remaining 3 1/2 green onions and set aside.

3. Add garlic, sliced green onions, sesame oil, eggs and ginger to food processor or high-speed blender with. Process until coarsely ground, then transfer to large mixing bowl.

4. Add ground meat and almond flour to bowl and mix well with hands or large wooden spoon. Roll mixture into golf ball sized meatballs with scoop or hands.

5. Place meatballs on prepared sheet pan. Bake for 15 - 20 minutes, until golden brown and cooked through.

6. For *Sauce*, peel and mince garlic. Add to small mixing bowl with fish sauce, vinegar, honey, oil and ginger. Mix well.

7. Remove meatballs from oven. Dip in *Sauce* with mini serving fork or toothpick and transfer to serving dish. Transfer remaining *Sauce* to serving dish.

8. Slice remaining 1/2 green onion. Sprinkle sesame seeds and reserved green onions over dish. Serve warm.

Chinese Orange Chicken

Prep Time: 10 minutes

Cook Time: 10 minutes

Servings: 2

INGREDIENTS

12 oz (3/4 lb) boneless skinless chicken

1/2 cup almond flour

1 teaspoon flax meal

1 cage-free egg

1 green onion (scallion)

1/4 teaspoon cayenne pepper

1/2 teaspoon paprika

1/2 teaspoon ground black pepper

1/2 teaspoon Celtic sea salt

Coconut oil (for cooking)

Water

Orange Sauce

3 oranges (or tangerines or Clementines)

2 tablespoons raw honey (or agave)

1 tablespoon tamari (or liquid aminos or coconut aminos)

1 small garlic clove

1/2 inch piece fresh ginger

1/4 teaspoon ground black pepper

Water

INSTRUCTIONS

1. For *Orange Sauce*, zest 2 oranges, *then* juice all oranges into small pot. Peel and mince garlic and ginger. Add to pot with honey, tamari and pepper. Add 1/2 cup water.

2. Heat small pot over medium heat and bring to simmer. Simmer until *Orange Sauce* is reduced by half, about 5 minutes. Stir frequently. Remove from heat and set aside.

3. Heat medium pan over medium-high heat. Lightly coat pan with coconut oil.

4. In a shallow dish, blend almond meal, flax meal, salt and spices.

5. Whisk egg and 1 teaspoon water in separate shallow dish.

6. Cut chicken into 1 inch pieces. Dip chicken into egg wash, then dredge in seasoned almond meal.

7. Carefully place coated chicken pieces into hot oil and fry about 2 - 3 minutes, until golden brown and cooked through. Turn with tongs halfway through cooking.

8. Drain cooked chicken on paper towel, then transfer to medium mixing bowl. Pour *Orange Sauce* over chicken and toss to coat. Transfer to serving dish.

9. Slice scallions and sprinkle over dish. Serve hot.

Sweet and Sour Chicken Bites

Prep Time: 15 minutes

Cook Time: 25 minutes

Servings: 2

INGREDIENTS

12 oz (3/4 lb) boneless skinless chicken

1 large cage-free egg

1/2 cup arrowroot powder

2 tablespoons tapioca flour (or arrowroot powder)

1 tablespoon coconut flour

2 tablespoons coconut aminos (or coconut vinegar or liquid aminos)

1 teaspoon garlic powder

1/2 teaspoon ground black pepper

1/2 teaspoon Celtic sea salt

Coconut oil (for cooking)

Sweet and Sour Sauce

3/4 cup pineapple juice

1/3 cup organic tomato sauce

1/4 cup raw honey (or agave or date butter)

1/4 cup coconut vinegar (or apple cider vinegar)

1 tablespoon tamari (or coconut aminos or liquid aminos)

1 tablespoon arrowroot powder (or tapioca flour)

1/4 inch piece fresh ginger

1/4 teaspoon allspice

1/4 teaspoon onion powder

1/2 teaspoon Celtic sea salt

Coconut oil (for cooking)

INSTRUCTIONS

1. For *Sweet and Sour Sauce*, peel and finely grate ginger. Add to food processor or high-speed blender with pineapple juice, tomato sauce, honey, vinegar, tamari, arrowroot, salt and spices. Process until smooth, about 1 minute.

2. Pour *Sweet and Sour Sauce* into small pot and heat over medium heat. Bring to simmer. Reduce heat to medium-low and cook until *Sweet and Sour Sauce* is reduced and thickened, about 10 - 15 minutes. Stir occasionally. Remove from heat and set aside.

3. Heat medium pan over medium-high heat. Coat pan with about 1/4 inch coconut oil.

4. In a shallow dish, blend coconut flour and tapioca flour, salt and spices. In small bowl, whisk together egg, arrowroot and coconut aminos.

5. Cut chicken into 1 inch pieces. Dip chicken in egg batter, then dredge in flour mixture.

6. Carefully place coated chicken pieces into hot oil and fry about 2 - 3 minutes, until golden brown and cooked through. Turn with tongs halfway through cooking.

7. Drain cooked chicken on paper towel, then transfer to serving dish. Transfer *Sweet and Sour Sauce* to serving dish.

8. Serve hot.

Asian Style Calamari

Prep Time: 15 minutes

Cook Time: 20 minutes

Servings: 4

INGREDIENTS

12 oz (3/4) medium whole squid (calamari)

2 cage-free eggs

1/4 cup almond flour

1/4 cup coconut flour

1/4 cup arrowroot powder

1/4 teaspoon Celtic sea salt

Water

Ginger Sauce

1 yellow onion

2 inch piece fresh ginger

1 lemon

1/2 cup coconut vinegar (or apple cider vinegar)

1/2 cup pure fish sauce (or tamari or coconut aminos)

1/2 cup tamari (or coconut aminos or liquid aminos)

INSTRUCTIONS

1. For *Ginger Sauce*, peel and chop ginger and onion. Add to food processor or high-speed blender and process until coarsely ground, about 1 minute. Add lemon juice, vinegar, fish sauce and tamari. Process until smooth, about 1 minute.

2. Pour mixture into small pot and heat over medium heat. Bring to simmer. Reduce heat to medium-low and cook until *Ginger Sauce* is reduced and thickened, about 10 - 15 minutes. Stir occasionally. Remove from heat and set aside. Then transfer to serving dish.

3. Have fishmonger clean squid. Or remove innards, clean and rinse squid yourself. Then cut into 1/3 inch rings, keeping tentacles intact.

4. Heat medium pan over medium-high heat. Coat pan with about 1/2 inch coconut oil.

5. Add arrowroot to shallow dish. Blend almond flour, coconut, flour and salt to separate shallow dish. Beat eggs and 1 tablespoon water in small mixing bowl or third shallow dish.

6. Dredge calamari rings and tentacles in arrowroot, shaking off excess. Transfer to dish for storage between steps.

7. Dip dusted squid into egg mixture, tossing gently to coat. Shake off excess and place back on dish.

8. Dredge dipped squid in flour mixture and carefully place directly into hot oil. Do not return to dish. Fry about 3 - 5 minutes, until golden brown and just cooked through. Tentacles cook slightly faster than rings. Turn half way through cooking with chopsticks or tongs.

9. Drain calamari on paper towel, then transfer to serving dish.

10. Serve hot with *Ginger Sauce*.

Triple Cashew Chicken

Prep Time: 10 minutes

Cook Time: 15 minutes

Servings: 4

INGREDIENTS

16 oz (1 lb) boneless, skinless chicken

1 cup raw cashews

1/4 cup cashew butter

1 cage-free egg

Pinch cayenne pepper (optional)

1/4 teaspoon Chinese 5-spice (optional)

1/4 teaspoon ground ginger

1/4 teaspoon garlic powder

1/2 teaspoon ground black pepper

1 teaspoon Celtic sea salt

Bacon fat or coconut oil (for cooking)

Water

INSTRUCTIONS

1. Heat large skillet or pan over medium-high heat. Add 1 - 2 tablespoons bacon fat or coconut oil to hot pan.
2. Add cashews to food processor or high-speed blender. Process until finely chopped or coarsely ground, about 1 minute. Transfer half of cashews to shallow dish.
3. Process remaining cashew until finely ground into flour, about 2 minutes. Transfer cashew flour to separate shallow dish.

4. Add cashew butter and egg to third shallow dish. Mix well to combine. Add enough water to reach saucy consistency.

5. Cut chicken into 1/2 inch strips. Dredge in cashew flour and toss to coat well. Then dip into egg mixture and toss to coat. Place chicken in chopped cashews and press to coat well.

6. Place chicken in hot oiled pan and cook about 1 - 2 minutes on each side, until golden brown and cooked through. Stir occasionally, careful to maintain coating.

7. Transfer cooked chicken to serving dish and serve hot.

Zucchini Noodle Pad Thai

Prep Time: 10 minutes

Cook Time: 15 minutes

Servings: 2

INGREDIENTS

12 oz (3/4 lb) boneless, skinless chicken breasts

2 cage-free eggs

1 large zucchini

1 large carrot

2 green onions (scallions)

3 small garlic cloves

1 shallot

1/2 teaspoon Celtic Sea salt

1/2 teaspoon ground black pepper

Bacon fat or coconut oil (for cooking)

Pad Thai Sauce

3 dried pitted dates

2 tablespoons pure fish sauce

2 tablespoons coconut aminos (liquid aminos or tamari)

1 tablespoon raw honey (or agave)

1 tablespoon apple cider vinegar

1 tablespoon fresh lime juice

1/3 teaspoon ground ginger

1/4 teaspoon cayenne pepper

Topping

1/4 cup raw cashews

Small bunch cilantro

1/2 lime

INGREDIENTS

1. For *Pad Thai Sauce*, add dates, fish sauce, coconut aminos, honey, vinegar, lime juice, ginger and pepper to food processor or high-speed blender. Process until smooth, about 1 minute. Set aside.

2. Use spiralizer, mandolin, vegetable peeler or grater to thinly slice zucchini and carrot. Add to medium bowl. Slice green onion and add to bowl. Set aside.

3. Peel and finely chop shallots and garlic. Whisk eggs in small mixing bowl. Cut chicken breasts into 1/2 inch pieces and season with salt and pepper.

4. Heat large skillet or wok over medium-high heat. Add 1 - 2 tablespoons bacon fat or coconut oil to hot pan.

5. Add chicken to hot oiled pan or wok and sauté about 2 minutes. Add shallots and garlic and sauté about 1 minute.

6. Add zucchini, carrot and scallions. Sauté until chicken is cooked through, about 2 minutes. Drain any excess liquid from pan and return to heat.

7. Push chicken and veggies aside and make well (opening) in center of pan. Pour whisked eggs into well and carefully scramble until fully cooked, about 2 minutes. Mix eggs into chicken and veggies.

8. Stir 2/3 of *Pad Thai Sauce* into chicken and veggie until combined. Transfer to serving dish. Transfer remaining *Pad Thai Sauce* to serving dish.

9. For *Topping*, finely chop cashews and cilantro and sprinkle over dish. Cut lime into wedges and serve with *Pad Thai*.
10. Serve immediately.

Mei Fun

Prep Time: 10 minutes

Cook Time: 10 minutes

Servings: 4

INSTRUCTIONS

1 package (12 oz) kelp noodles

2 cage-free eggs

2 celery stalks

1 cup cabbage (shredded or chopped)

1/2 large green pepper

1/2 large onion (yellow or white)

8 green onions (scallions)

2 garlic cloves

1 1/2 tablespoons curry powder

1 lemon

Coconut oil (for cooking)

Sauce

1/4 cup pure fish sauce

1 tablespoon tamari (or coconut aminos or liquid aminos)

1 teaspoon raw honey (or agave)

1 teaspoon tomato paste

Pinch all spice

Pinch onion powder

DIRECTIONS

1. Drain and rinse kelp noodles. Add to medium bowl and soak in water and lemon juice for 5 minutes.

2. Heat large skillet or wok over high heat. Add 2 tablespoon oil to hot pan.

3. For *Sauce*, add fish sauce, tamari, honey, tomato paste, allspice and onion powder to small mixing bowl. Stir to combine. Set aside.

4. Remove stems, seed and veins from pepper, then slice. Peel onion and slice. Shred cabbage. Thinly slice celery. Set aside.

5. Peel garlic and mince. Thinly slice half of green onions. Chop remaining green onions. Whisk eggs in small mixing bowl.

6. Add whisked eggs to hot oiled pan and scramble until set, about 1 - 2 minutes. Transfer to small dish and set aside.

7. Add 2 tablespoons oil to hot pan. Add minced garlic to pan and sauté until aromatic, about 1 minute. Add onion, pepper, celery, cabbage and chopped green onions to pan. Sauté about 2 minutes.

8. Drain and add kelp noodles, curry powder and sliced scallions to pan. Sauté 1 minute. Add *Sauce* and scrambled eggs. Sauté about 1 minute to warm through.

9. Transfer to serving dish and serve hot.

Fresh Noodle Chicken Chow Fun

Prep Time: 20 minutes

Cook Time: 20 minutes

Servings: 2

INGREDIENTS

8 oz (1/2 lb) boneless, skinless chicken

3/4 cup chicken broth

1/4 cup pure fish sauce (or tamari)

1/2 cup bean sprouts

1 celery stalk

4 button mushrooms

3.5 oz (1/2 can) sliced water chestnuts

3 teaspoons arrowroot flour

1 teaspoon Chinese 5-spice

Bacon fat or coconut oil (for cooking)

Noodles

1/2 cup almond flour

1/2 cup arrowroot powder

1/2 cup tapioca flour

1 cage-free egg

2 cage-free egg yolks

1 tablespoon coconut oil (or sesame oil)

1 teaspoon Celtic sea salt

INSTRUCTIONS

1. Bring medium pot of lightly salted water to a boil.

2. For *Noodles*, sift almond flour, tapioca flour, 1/3 cup arrow powder and salt into medium mixing bowl. Make well in center of flour mixture and add egg and yolks. Start to whisk eggs into flour in circular motion with a fork until dough pulls together.

3. Dust cutting board with half of remaining arrowroot powder. Turn dough out onto cutting board and knead for 5 minutes, until smooth. Add 1 tablespoon coconut oil or almond flour if dough is too dry or too moist or sticky.

4. Dust cutting board with remaining arrowroot powder. Roll dough into rectangular shape with a rolling pin to about 1/8 inch thick. Cut pasta sheet into long strips with pizza cutter or sharp knife.

5. Or run pasta through pasta machine several times to reach desired consistency. Then use cutting attachment to cut pasta into desired style.

6. Place cut pasta in boiling water one portion at a time for 2 - 3 minutes to prevent sticking. Drain pasta in colander. Set aside.

7. Heat medium pan or wok over high heat. Add 2 tablespoons bacon fat or coconut oil to hot pan.

8. Slice celery and mushrooms. Cut chicken into 1/4 inch strips.

9. Add chicken to hot oiled pan and sauté about 2 minutes. Stir frequently. Transfer to dish and set aside.

10. Add celery, mushrooms, water chestnuts and bean sprouts to hot pan. Sauté about 1 minute. Then add chicken stock, fish sauce, arrowroot and five-spice. Sauté another minute, until liquid thickens and reduces slightly.

11. Add chicken back to pan and sauté 1 - 2 minutes, until chicken is cooked through. Add *Noodles* and sauté to heat through, about 1 minute.

12. Transfer to serving dish and serve hot.

Thai-Style Coconut Chicken

Prep Time: 10 minutes

Cook Time: 15 minutes

Servings: 4

INGREDIENTS

16 oz (1 lb) boneless, skinless chicken

3 cage-free egg whites

1 cup flaked or shredded coconut

1/4 teaspoon ground ginger

1/2 teaspoon garlic powder

1/2 teaspoon ground white pepper (or ground black pepper)

1 teaspoon Celtic sea salt

Coconut oil (for cooking)

Coconut Glaze

1/3 cup raw honey (or agave)

1/3 cup coconut milk

1/4 cup flaked or shredded coconut

1 tablespoon fresh lime juice

1/4 teaspoon ground ginger

Pinch Celtic sea salt

Water

INSTRUCTIONS

1. Preheat oven to 425 degrees F. Line sheet pan with parchment paper. Or place oven-safe wire rack over sheet pan.

2. Add coconut to shallow dish. Set aside.

3. Add egg whites, ginger, garlic, salt and pepper to large mixing bowl. Beat with hand mixer or whisk until light and fluffy, about 2 - 4 minutes.

4. Cut chicken into 1 inch cubes and add to egg whites. Toss to coat.

5. Let excess egg white drain from chicken, then add to coconut flakes. Toss to coat. Return chicken to egg whites, then coconut flakes again. Press chicken into flaked coconut and coat well.

6. Place coated chicken on prepared sheet pan. Brush lightly with coconut oil.

7. Place in oven and bake for about 5 minutes. Turn chicken over and brush with coconut oil. Bake about 5 minutes, until coconut is golden brown and chicken is cooked through are bright pink.

8. For *Coconut Sauce*, add honey, coconut milk, shredded coconut, lime juice, ginger and salt to small pot. Add water to reach desired glaze consistency, if necessary.

9. Heat over medium heat and bring to simmer. Remove from heat and transfer to large mixing bowl.

10. Remove chicken from oven and add to bowl. Toss with *Coconut Sauce*.

11. Transfer to serving dish and serve hot.

Sesame Chicken

Prep Time: 10 minutes

Cook Time: 20 minutes

Servings: 2

INGREDIENTS

12 oz (3/4 lb) boneless skinless chicken

1/4 cup almond flour

1/4 cup arrowroot powder

1 large cage-free egg white

2 teaspoon sesame seeds

1/4 teaspoon cayenne pepper

1/2 teaspoon garlic powder

1/2 teaspoon ground black pepper

1/2 teaspoon Celtic sea salt

Coconut oil (for cooking)

Garlic Sauce

1/2 yellow onion

1/2 lemon

6 garlic cloves

1/4 inch piece fresh ginger

1/4 cup date butter (or raw honey or agave)

2 tablespoons pure fish sauce

2 tablespoons coconut aminos (or tamar or liquid aminos)

2 tablespoons tamari (or liquid aminos or coconut aminos)

1/4 teaspoon ground black pepper

Water

INSTRUCTIONS

1. For *Garlic Sauce*, peel onions, garlic and ginger. Roughly chop and add to food processor or high-speed blender. Add date butter, fish sauce, coconut aminos, tamari and black pepper. Process until smooth.

2. Add sesame seeds to small pot. Heat over medium heat and toast about 2 minutes. Stir constantly. Transfer to small bowl and set aside.

3. Pour *Garlic Sauce* into pot and cook until onions and date butter until caramelized and garlic is fragrant, about 5 minutes. Stir frequently.

4. Add enough water to create saucy consistency. Stir frequently and bring to simmer. Simmer until *Garlic Sauce* is reduced by half and browned, about 5 minutes. Remove from heat and set aside.

5. Heat medium pan over medium-high heat. Coat pan with about 1/4 inch coconut oil.

6. In a shallow dish, blend almond meal, arrowroot powder, salt and spices.

7. Beat egg whites in small mixing bowl with hand mixer or whisk until light and frothy, about 2 - 4 minutes.

8. Cut chicken into 1 inch pieces. Dip chicken in egg whites, then dredge in seasoned flour mixture.

9. Carefully place coated chicken pieces into hot oil and fry about 2 - 3 minutes, until golden brown and cooked through. Turn with tongs halfway through cooking.

10. Drain cooked chicken on paper towel, then transfer to medium mixing bowl. Pour *Garlic Sauce* and 1 teaspoon toasted sesame seeds over chicken and toss to coat. Transfer to serving dish.

11. Sprinkle remaining toasted sesame seeds over dish. Serve hot.

Classic General Tso's Chicken

Prep Time: 10 minutes

Cook Time: 15 minutes

Servings: 2

INGREDIENTS

12 oz (3/4 lb) boneless skinless chicken

1/4 cup almond flour

1/4 cup arrowroot powder

1 large cage-free egg white

1 small green onion (scallion)

1/2 teaspoon red pepper flakes

1/2 teaspoon garlic powder

1/2 teaspoon paprika

1/2 teaspoon ground black pepper

1/2 teaspoon Celtic sea salt

Coconut oil (for cooking)

Sauce

3/4 cup water

3 teaspoons arrowroot powder (or tapioca flour)

2 tablespoons date butter (or raw honey or agave)

2 tablespoons coconut vinegar (or apple cider vinegar)

3 tablespoons coconut aminos (or liquid aminos or tamari)

1 teaspoon sesame oil

1 teaspoon coconut oil

1 teaspoon almond butter

2 garlic cloves

1/2 inch piece fresh ginger

1 red chili pepper

1/4 teaspoon Chinese 5-spice

Pinch ground black pepper

Pinch Celtic sea salt

INSTRUCTIONS

1. For *Sauce*, peel garlic and ginger. Add to food processor or high-speed blender with water, arrowroot powder, date butter, vinegar, coconut aminos, sesame oil, coconut oil, almind butter, chili pepper, salt and spices. Process until smooth.

2. Pour *Sauce* into small pot and heat over medium heat. Stir frequently and bring to simmer. Cook until *Sauce* is reduced and thickened, about 3 - 4 minutes. Remove from heat and set aside.

3. Heat medium pan over medium-high heat. Coat pan with about 1/4 inch coconut oil.

4. In a shallow dish, blend almond meal, arrowroot powder, salt and spices.

5. Beat egg whites in small mixing bowl with hand mixer or whisk until light and frothy, about 2 - 4 minutes.

6. Cut chicken into 1 inch pieces. Dip chicken in egg whites, then dredge in seasoned flour mixture.

7. Carefully place coated chicken pieces into hot oil and fry about 2 - 3 minutes, until golden brown and cooked through. Turn with tongs halfway through cooking.

8. Drain cooked chicken on paper towel, then transfer to medium mixing bowl. Pour *Sauce* and red pepper flakes over chicken and toss to coat. Transfer to serving dish.

9. Slice green onion and sprinkle over dish. Serve hot.

Indian Egg Fried Rice

Prep Time: 10 minutes

Cook Time: 15 minutes

Servings: 2

INGREDIENTS

1/2 head cauliflower

4 cage-free eggs

1 small carrot

1/2 red bell pepper

1/2 yellow bell pepper

1/4 onion (yellow or white)

2 small green onions (scallions)

2 tablespoons pure fish sauce (or coconut aminos or liquid aminos)

1 tablespoon coconut aminos (or coconut vinegar or liquid aminos)

1 teaspoon raw honey (or date butter or agave)

1 teaspoon sesame oil (optional)

1 large garlic clove

1/2 piece fresh ginger

1/2 teaspoon red pepper flake

Celtic sea salt, to taste

Bacon fat or coconut oil (for cooking)

Water

INSTRUCTIONS

1. Cut cauliflower into florets and add to food processor with shredding attachment to rice. Or finely mince cauliflower. Set aside.

2. Heat medium pan or wok over high heat. Lightly coat with bacon fat or coconut oil.

3. Whisk eggs in medium mixing bowl. Set aside.

4. Remove stems, seeds and veins from bell peppers, then julienne (thinly slice). Finely dice carrot. Slice green onions. Peel and mince garlic, ginger and onion.

5. Add red pepper flakes to hot oiled pan. Sauté until just cooked fragrant, about 30 seconds. Add garlic, ginger and onion and sauté about 1 minute.

6. Add cauliflower to hot pan. Sauté about 5 minutes, until cauliflower is golden and a bit softened.

7. Add carrot, peppers and 1/2 green onions. Cook another 2 - 5 minutes, until cauliflower is cooked through. Add a few tablespoons of water and cover with lid to steam, if desired.

8. Push veggies aside and make well (opening) in center of pan. Pour whisked eggs into well in center and carefully scramble until fully cooked, about 2 minutes. Mix eggs into veggies.

9. Remove from heat and transfer to serving dish. Spprinkle remaining green onions over dish and serve hot.

Chicken and Cashew Stir-Fry

Prep Time: 5 minutes

Cook Time: 10 minutes

Servings: 2

INGREDIENTS

12 oz (3/4 lb) boneless skinless chicken

1/2 cup raw cashews

1/2 small onion (white or yellow)

1/2 red bell pepper

1/2 green bell pepper

1 small celery stalk

2 tablespoons tamari (or coconut aminos or apple cider vinegar)

1 teaspoon raw honey (or agave or date butter)

1 garlic clove

1/2 inch piece fresh ginger

1/4 teaspoon ground black pepper

1/2 teaspoon Celtic sea salt

Bacon fat or coconut oil (for cooking)

INSTRUCTIONS

1. Heat large pan or wok over medium heat. Lightly coat with bacon fat or coconut oil.

2. Peel and mince garlic and ginger. Remove seeds, stems and veins from peppers, then roughly chop. Dice carrot. Slice celery.

3. Roughly chop chicken and season with salt and pepper.

4. Add garlic and ginger to hot oiled pan or wok. Sauté about 1 minute, until fragrant. Add seasoned chicken add sauté until browned, about 2 minutes. Transfer chicken to small bowl and set aside.

5. Add veggies to hot oiled pan. Sauté until tender and lightly browned, about 2 minutes. Add tamari, honey and cashews. Sauté until veggies are just cooked, but still crisp.

6. Add chicken back to pan and heat until just cooked through, about 2 minutes.

7. Transfer to serving dish and serve hot.

Spicy Beef and Broccoli

Prep Time: 20 minutes

Cook Time: 10 minutes

Servings: 2

INGREDIENTS

12 oz (3/4 lb) beef sirloin

1/2 head broccoli

2 carrots

1 tablespoon tamari (or coconut aminos)

1 tablespoon dry sherry (or pure fish sauce or apple cider vinegar)

1 garlic clove

1/2 inch piece fresh ginger

1/2 teaspoon sesame seeds (optional)

Coconut oil (for cooking)

Sauce

1 tablespoon Asian chili paste

3 teaspoons tamari (or coconut aminos)

3 teaspoons chicken broth (or beef broth)

3 teaspoons dry sherry (or pure fish sauce or apple cider vinegar)

1 teaspoon raw honey (or agave)

1/2 teaspoon arrowroot flour

1/2 teaspoon sesame oil

2 garlic cloves

1/4 teaspoon fresh ground black pepper

INSTRUCTIONS

1. Cut beef against the grain into thin slices. Add to small mixing with tamari and sherry. And toss to coat. Set aside to marinate for 20 minutes.

2. For Sauce, peel and mince garlic. Add to small mixing bowl with chili paste, tamari, broth, sherry, honey, arrowroot, sesame oil and pepper. Mix to combine. Set aside.

3. Roughly chop broccoli into pieces. Slice carrots diagonally. Peel and mince garlic and ginger. Set aside.

4. Heat medium pan or wok over medium heat. Add 1 tablespoon coconut oil to hot pan.

5. Add marinated beef to hot pan in single layer. Let sear 1 minute on each side, undisturbed. Transfer to medium dish and set aside.

6. Add 1 tablespoon coconut oil to hot pan. Add garlic and ginger and sauté about 1 minute. Add broccoli and carrots. Sauté until lightly browned and softened, about 3 - 4 minutes. Stir frequently.

7. Add beef back to pan with *Sauce* and sesame seeds. Sauté until veggies are tender and beef is cooked through, about 2 minutes.

8. Transfer to serving dish and serve hot.

Tender Grilled Korean Beef

Prep Time: 5 minutes*

Cook Time: 20 minutes

Servings: 4

INGREDIENTS

16 oz (1 lb) beef sirloin

1 medium carrot

1 green onion (scallion)

1/2 onion (yellow or white)

3 tablespoons tamari (or coconut aminos or liquid aminos)

1 tablespoon sesame oil

1 tablespoon sesame seeds

1 teaspoon raw honey (or agave)

1 garlic clove

1/2 teaspoon ground black pepper

1/2 teaspoon Celtic sea salt

INSTRUCTIONS

1. Peel and mince garlic. Add to large kitchen bag or medium container with lid with tamari, sesame oil, sesame seeds, honey, salt and pepper. Mix to combine.

2. Peel and chop onions. Julienne (thinly slice lengthwise) carrots. Chop green onion. Thinly slice beef. Add to container and toss or mix well to coat. Set aside in refrigerate at least 3 hours to marinate.

3. Heat outdoor grill to high heat.

4. Drain beef and vegetables from marinade and place on large sheet of aluminum foil. Fold foil over meat and veggies to make sealed packet.
5. Place on grill and cook 20 minutes, for about medium-well doneness.
6. Carefully remove packet from grill and place on cutting board. Carefully open one end of packet and release steam for about 1 minute. Open packet and transfer meat and veggies to serving dish.
7. Serve hot.

Stir-Fried Mongolian Beef

Prep Time: 15 minutes

Cook Time: 10 minutes

Servings: 2

INGREDIENTS

16 oz (1 lb) beef flank steak

1/4 cup arrowroot powder

2 large green onions

Coconut oil (for cooking)

Sauce

1/3 - 1/2 cup date butter (or raw honey or agave)

1/4 cup pure fish sauce

1/4 cup tamari (or liquid aminos or coconut aminos)

1/4 inch piece ginger

2 garlic cloves

1/2 cup water

Bacon fat or coconut oil (for cooking)

INSTRUCTIONS

1. Add arrowroot to shallow dish. Cut steak against the grain into 1/4 inch pieces. Dip each piece into arrowroot and lightly coat on both sides. Set aside for 10 minutes.

2. Heat large pan or wok over medium heat. Add about 1 cup coconut oil to hot pan.

3. Add coated beef to hot oil and cook for about 3 - 4 minutes, gently can carefully stirring constantly. Use slotted spoon to remove beef from oil and drain on paper towels. Set aside.

4. For *Sauce*, heat medium pan over medium heat. Add 1 tablespoon bacon fat or coconut oil to hot pan.

5. Peel and finely grate ginger and garlic. Add to medium pan and sauté until just golden and aromatic, about 30 seconds. Add fish sauce, tamari, date butter and water. Stir and cook until reduced and thickened, about 2 - 3 minutes.

6. Slice green onions on a diagonal into 1 inch pieces. Add to sauce with beef and sauté about 1 minute.

7. Transfer to serving dish and serve hot.

Asian Orange Roasted Duck

Prep Time: 40 minutes

Cook Time: 2 hours

Servings: 4

INGREDIENTS

1 (6 lb) whole duck (innards removed)

2 oranges (or tangerines or Clementines)

2 inch piece fresh ginger

1 tablespoon Chinese 5-spice

1 teaspoon fresh cracked black peppercorns (or peppercorn medley)

1 tablespoon Celtic sea salt

Water

Orange Glaze

4 oranges (or tangerines or Clementines)

2 cups water

3 tablespoons raw honey (or agave)

3 tablespoons tamari (or liquid aminos or coconut aminos)

INSTRUCTIONS

1. Rinse duck thoroughly and pat dry with paper towel. Pierce all over with tip of paring knife or fork, then place in heat-safe container just large enough to fit duck.

2. For *Orange Glaze*, slice 2 oranges into 1/4 inch slices and add to medium pot with water, sweetener and tamari. Juice remaining 2 oranges into pot. Heat over medium heat and bring to boil, stirring

occasionally. Reduce to medium-low heat and simmer until reduced by half, about 10 minutes.

3. Carefully pour or ladle *Orange Glaze* over duck in container. Set aside to marinate about 30 minutes.

4. Preheat oven to 325 degrees F. Set rack back into roasting pan.

5. Remove duck from container and discard *Orange Glaze*. Rub duck with salt, pepper and 5-spice. Place rack in roasting pan.

6. Quarter oranges. Peel and slice ginger into 1/4 in slices. Stuff duck with oranges and ginger. Secure cavity closed with toothpicks, skewers or kitchen twine.

7. Pour 1 cup water into pan. Place in middle of oven and bake for 90 minutes. Increase oven to 450 degrees F and roast about 25 - 30 minutes, until skin is dark brown and crisp, and internal temperature reaches at least 170 degrees F.

8. Remove from oven and let rest about 10 minutes.

9. Carve duck and serve warm.

Braised Spare Ribs

Prep Time: 15 minutes

Cook Time: 3 hours 15 minutes

Servings: 4

INGREDIENTS

5 lbs beef short ribs

1 cup pure fish sauce

1/4 cup coconut vinegar (or apple cider vinegar)

1/4 cup tamari (or coconut aminos)

1/4 - 1/2 cup raw honey (or agave)

6 - 8 green onions

1 lemongrass stalk

3 garlic cloves

1 inch piece fresh ginger

1 orange

1 small lemon

1 teaspoon sesame seeds

3/4 teaspoon red pepper flakes

Water

DIRECTIONS

1. Preheat oven to 350 degrees F.
2. Cut ribs into portions. Cut green onions in half. Slice white bottoms and reserve green tops. Peel ginger. Peel and smash garlic. Split and smash lemon grass.

3. Add rib portions, fish sauce, honey, green onions, lemongrass, ginger garlic, red pepper, juice of 1/2 orange and water to wide pot. Ribs should be submerged.

4. Cover and back about 3 hours, until meat is tender and falling off the bone. Remove ribs from braising liquid and cover to keep warm.

5. Increase oven to 425 degrees F.

6. Drain fat off braising liquid and discard. Add remaining liquid to medium pan with tamari. Heat over medium-high heat and bring to a boil.

7. Simmer about 5 minutes, until reduced. Strain liquid through strainer or sieve to remove solids. Return to pan. Juice remaining 1/2 orange and lemon into pan. Stir to combine.

8. Add ribs back to pot and coat with reduction Bake for 10 minutes, until heated through and glazed. Transfer to serving dish.

9. Slice reserved green onion tops. Sprinkle green onions and sesame seeds over dish. Serve warm.

Coconut Lime Thai Steamed Mussels

Prep Time: 10 minutes

Cook Time: 10

Servings: 2

INGREDIENTS

2.5 lbs fresh mussels

1/2 can (about 6.5 oz) coconut milk

3 tablespoons dry white wine (or tamari or coconut vinegar)

2 teaspoons Thai red curry paste

1/2 tablespoon pure fish sauce

1/2 tablespoon raw honey (or agave)

2 garlic cloves

1 bunch fresh cilantro

2 limes

INSTRUCTIONS

1. Have fishmonger clean mussels. Or scrub mussels and remove the beards with pliers yourself, if necessary.
2. Juice limes into large pot with lid. Peel and mince garlic. Add to pot with coconut milk, wine, curry paste, fish sauce and honey. Heat over high heat and bring to boil. Stir frequently.
3. Simmer for 1 minute, then add mussels. Cover with lid and cook until mussels open, about 5 - 8 minutes. Sir occasionally.
4. Remove from heat. Chop cilantro and toss with mussels.
5. Transfer mussels and liquid to serving dish. Serve hot.

Asian Mustard Baked Salmon

Prep Time: 5 minutes

Cook Time: 20 minutes

Servings: 2

INGREDIENTS

2 (8 oz) salmon fillets (deboned, skin-on)

2 cups bok choy or Chinese broccoli (roughly chopped)

1/2 teaspoon sesame seeds

Parchment paper

Kitchen twine

Mustard Sauce

1/4 cup pure fish sauce

2 tablespoons Chinese hot mustard (or Dijon or spicy brown mustard)

1 tablespoon raw honey (or agave)

1 tablespoon tamari (or coconut aminos)

1 tablespoon coconut oil

1/2 lime

1 garlic clove

1/2 inch piece fresh ginger

INSTRUCTIONS

1. Preheat oven to 400 degrees F. Place large sheet pan on bottom rack of oven. Prepare large sheet of parchment.

2. For *Mustard Sauce*, peel and mince garlic and ginger. Add to small mixing bowl with fish sauce, mustard, honey, tamari, coconut oil and lime juice. Mix to combine. Set aside.

3. Chop bok choy or Chinese broccoli and place in the middle of parchment sheet.

4. Place salmon fillets skin-side down over veggies. Brush well with *Mustard Sauce*. Transfer remaining mustard sauce to serving dish.

5. Gather edges of parchment up over salmon and tie tightly with kitchen twine to form sealed pouch.

6. Place pouch directly on hot baking sheet in hot oven. Bake for 20 minutes.

7. Remove from oven and carefully open pouch to release steam. Transfer veggies and salmon to serving dish.

8. Serve hot with remaining *Mustard Sauce*.

Coconut Egg Custard Tartlets

Prep Time: 25 minutes

Cook Time: 20 minutes

Servings: 4

INGREDIENTS

Crust

1 1/4 cups almond flour

1/3 cup coconut oil

3 teaspoons raw honey (or agave)

1/2 teaspoon vanilla

Filling

2 (13 oz) cans full-fat coconut milk

8 cage-free eggs

1/4 cup arrowroot powder

1/4 cup raw honey (or agave)

1 teaspoon vanilla

Pinch Celtic sea salt

INSTRUCTIONS

1. Preheat oven to 350 degrees F. Lightly coat 4 small or 12 mini tart pans with coconut oil.

2. For *Crust*, add almond flour, coconut oil, honey and vanilla to small mixing bowl. Mix well until soft but crumbly dough comes together.

3. Press dough into tart shells and set aside.

4. Add coconut milk, arrowroot powder, sweetener, vanilla and salt to medium pot. Heat pot over medium heat and bring to a boil. Set aside to cool about 10 minutes.

5. Whisk eggs well in medium mixing bowl. Slowly whisk cooled coconut milk into eggs, careful not to scramble.

6. Strain mixture through strainer or sieve into separate bowl.

7. Pour strained mixture into tart shells and bake for 15 - 20 minutes, until filling is golden brown and set in the center.

8. Remove from oven and let cool at least 5 minutes. Remove from pans and transfer to serving dish.

9. Serve warm. Or let cool completely and serve room temperature.

Snacks Cookbook

Spicy Sweet Potato Brittle

Prep time: 10 minutes

Cook time: 30 minutes

INGREDIENTS

3 sweet potatoes

¼ cup extra virgin olive oil

¼ tsp Celtic sea salt

¼ tsp smoked paprika

INSTRUCTIONS

1. Preheat oven to 500 degrees.

2. Peel the potatoes and cut them into small wedges. In a large bowl, combine potato wedges, extra virgin olive oil, Celtic sea salt and smoked paprika. Mix well until all wedges are coated in all ingredients.

3. Place on a baking sheet and bake for 30 minutes, turning once halfway through, and continue cooking until they are well browned.

4. Remove from oven and let cool. Serve.

Celery with Baby Carrots

Prep time: 3 minutes

INGREDIENTS

2 tbsp organic Tahini

1 tsp cinnamon

½ cup baby carrots

1 stalk celery

INSTRUCTIONS

1. Slice the celery stalk into small pieces, about the size of the baby carrots.

2. In a very small bowl, mix the tahini and cinnamon together.

3. Serve. Eat by dipping the vegetables in the tahini/cinnamon mix.

Wheat Free Fruit Cookies

Prep time: 20 minutes

Cook time: 12 hours

INGREDIENTS

2 large bananas

2 lbs strawberries

INSTRUCTIONS

1. Cut the bananas into slices, about ⅛ to ¼ inch thick. Slice the tops of the strawberries and place each strawberry top over each banana slice.

2. Place it onto a dehydrator sheet and place in a dehydrator at 135 degrees for 12 hours.

3. Remove from dehydrator and serve.

Wheat Free Cashew Coconut Balls

Prep time: 15 minutes

INGREDIENTS

½ cup organic cashew butter

⅓ cup flaked coconut

2 tbsp organic maple syrup

¼ tsp cinnamon

INSTRUCTIONS

1. In a bowl, combine all the ingredients and mix well.

2. Separate into small balls and roll them together in your hands. Place the balls in the fridge for 20 minutes, or in the freezer to make them feel thicker.

3. Serve.

Cool Berry Drink

Prep time: 5 minutes

INGREDIENTS

¼ cup coconut milk

1 banana

1 cup strawberries

½ cup ice cubes

INSTRUCTIONS

1. Remove stems from strawberries.

2. Combine all the ingredients in a blender and blend until pureed.

3. Serve.

Raspberry Blend

Prep time: 5 minutes

INGREDIENTS

¼ cup coconut milk

1 banana

½ cup raspberries

½ cup peaches

½ cup ice cubes

INSTRUCTIONS

1. Remove pits from peaches.

2. Combine all the ingredients in a blender and blend until pureed.

3. Serve.

Icy Blueberry Delight

Prep time: 5 minutes

INGREDIENTS

¼ cup coconut milk

1 cup blueberries

½ cup plums

½ cup raspberries

½ cup ice cubes

INSTRUCTIONS

1. Remove pits from plums.

2. Combine all the ingredients in a blender and blend until pureed.

3. Serve.

Strawberry Blend

Prep time: 5 minutes

INGREDIENTS

¼ cup coconut milk

1 banana

½ cup mango

½ cup pineapple

½ cup ice cubes

INSTRUCTIONS

1. Remove stems from strawberries.

2. Combine all the ingredients in a blender and blend until pureed.

3. Serve.

Chunked Apples

Prep time: 10 minutes

Cook time: 10-15 minutes

INGREDIENTS

1 cup grapes

1 tsp arrowroot

½ cup water

3 large apples

INSTRUCTIONS

1. Boil water in a small saucepan.

2. Add the grapes to the water and boil until soft, about 2-3 minutes.

3. Cool the mixture; blend it and then strain, removing excess water.

4. In a pan, combine arrowroot, ½ cup water, and grape mixture.

5. Simmer until the mixture turns slightly thick and remove from heat.

6. Slice the apples in half and hollow out a decent portion surrounding the core.

7. Place an equal amount of grape mixture into the hollowed portion of each apple chunk.

8. Serve.

Baked Cauliflower

Prep time:

Cook time:

INGREDIENTS

1 head of cauliflower

3 tbsp extra virgin olive oil

¼ tsp Celtic sea salt

INSTRUCTIONS

1. Preheat oven to 425 degrees.

2. Cut the head of cauliflower down to smaller florets, about an inch or so in length.

3. In a large bowl, combine cauliflower, extra virgin olive oil and Celtic sea salt and mix.

4. Place the cauliflower on a baking sheet and roast for 1 hour. Turn the pieces 4 times during baking at 15 minute intervals.

5. Remove from oven and let cool. Serve.

Almond & Banana Bar

Prep time: 10 minutes

INGREDIENTS

1 banana

¼ cup almond butter

1 tbsp organic maple syrup

INSTRUCTIONS

1. Slice a banana horizontally to make 10 separate pieces.

2. Lay the pieces on a plate and place a dollop of almond butter between each piece, pressing together afterward.

3. Drizzle with organic maple syrup and serve.

Black Pepper & Kale Chips

Prep time: 15 minutes

Cook time: 10-15 minutes

INGREDIENTS

1 handful baby kale greens

¼ tsp garlic powder

2 tbsp coconut oil

¼ tsp Celtic sea salt

¼ tsp ground black pepper

INSTRUCTIONS

1. Preheat oven to 350 degrees.

2. In a large bowl, combine 2 tbsp melted coconut oil with kale greens, garlic powder, Celtic sea salt and ground black pepper. Mix well.

3. Line a baking sheet with parchment paper and place kale on it. Bake until the edges of the kale are browned, 10-15 minutes.

4. Remove from oven and cool. Serve.

Chocó Raisins

Prep time: 30 minutes

INGREDIENTS

1 cup raisins

two 1.4 oz bars of Enjoy Life Boom Choco Boom Dark Chocolate

INSTRUCTIONS

1. Boil water in a large saucepan. Cover the saucepan with a mesh top and place a small saucepan on top. Place the chocolate bars in the small saucepan and use the steam to melt them.

2. In a bowl, combine melted chocolate and raisins.

3. Place raisins on a wax paper sheet and place them in the freezer for 15 minutes to harden.

4. Serve.

Creamy Raspberry

Prep time: 30 minutes

INGREDIENTS

1 cup raspberries

coconut milk (amount will vary)

two 1.4 oz bars of Enjoy Life Boom Choco Boom Dark Chocolate

INSTRUCTIONS

1. Boil water in a large saucepan. Cover the saucepan with a mesh top and place a small saucepan on top. Place the chocolate bars in the small saucepan and use the steam to melt them.

2. Place a sheet of wax paper over a baking sheet and tape it down so it doesn't move. For each raspberry, place a small dollop of melted chocolate on a piece of wax paper, and place a raspberry on top of each dollop. Pour coconut milk into each raspberry, enough to slightly overfill each one. Top each raspberry with melted chocolate.

3. Carefully place the wax paper sheet in the freezer for 15 minutes to harden.

4. Serve

Mixed Fruit Drizzle

Prep time: 5 minutes

INGREDIENTS

1 banana

½ cup blueberries

2 tbsp coconut flakes

1 tbsp organic maple syrup

INSTRUCTIONS

1. Slice the banana.

2. In a serving bowl, combine banana, blueberries and coconut flakes.

   Mix well and drizzle with organic maple syrup.

3. Serve.

Fruits Blend

Prep time: 10 minutes

Cook time: 10 minutes

INGREDIENTS

Blueberry Sauce

1 cup blueberries

1 tbsp arrowroot

1 tbsp lemon juice

¼ tsp cinnamon

½ cup water

Fruits

1 banana

½ cup strawberries

INSTRUCTIONS

1. In a saucepan, combine blueberries, ½ cup water, arrowroot, cinnamon and lemon juice over medium heat. Simmer lightly until thick and remove from heat.

2. Slice banana and chop strawberries.

3. In a bowl, combine banana, strawberries, and blueberry sauce and mix.

4. Serve.

Broccoli Fries

Prep time: 15 minutes

Cook time: 20 minutes

INGREDIENTS

1 large bunch of broccoli

2 tbsp extra virgin olive oil

1 tbsp garlic powder

¼ tsp Celtic sea salt

INSTRUCTIONS

1. Preheat oven to 450 degrees. Cut the broccoli into florets.

2. In a large bowl, mix broccoli florets, extra virgin olive oil, garlic powder and Celtic sea salt.

3. Spread the broccoli over a baking sheet and roast for 20 minutes until the edges are crispy.

4. Remove from oven and let cool. Serve.

Nuts & Raisin Bars

Prep time: 5 minutes

INGREDIENTS

1 cup cashews

1 cup raisins

¼ tsp cinnamon

⅓ cup shredded coconut

INSTRUCTIONS

1. In a food processor, combine almonds, raisins and cinnamon, and process into a thick butter.

2. Add the coconut flakes and pulse for 15 seconds.

3. Place the mixture on a piece of wax paper and form it into a square. Place this in the freezer for 20 minutes.

4. Cut the square into appropriately-sized pieces. Serve.

Orange Nutmeg Treat

Prep time: 3 minutes

Cook time: 25 minutes

INGREDIENTS

1 gallon organic apple cider

2 cinnamon sticks

2 oranges

½ tsp nutmeg

1 tbsp whole cloves

INSTRUCTIONS

1. Slice oranges into at least 6 pieces each.

2. Combine all ingredients in a large saucepan and bring slowly to a boil, then immediately reduce heat and simmer lightly for 20 minutes.

3. Remove from heat and keep warm. Serve.

Rich Mixed Fruit Creamy Salad

Prep time: 5 minutes

INGREDIENTS

⅓ cup coconut milk

1 banana

¼ cup mango

¼ cup pineapple

¼ cup kiwi

INSTRUCTIONS

1. Combine all the ingredients in a blender. Blend until pureed.

2. Serve.

On the Go Cookbook

Strawberry Breakfast Pastry

Prep Time: 25 minutes

Cook Time: 20 minutes

Servings: 4

INSTRUCTIONS

Crust

2 cups almond flour

2 cage-free eggs

1/4 cup coconut oil (or ghee, cacao butter or coconut butter, softened)

1 tablespoon date butter (or honey or agave)

1/4 teaspoon baking soda

1/4 teaspoon vanilla

1/2 teaspoon Celtic sea salt

Filling

2 cups chopped strawberries (about 3/4 pint whole strawberries) (fresh or frozen)

2 tablespoons raw honey (or agave)

1/2 teaspoon vanilla

1/4 teaspoon Celtic sea salt

INSTRUCTIONS

1. Preheat oven to 400 degrees. Line sheet pan with parchment or baking mat. Cover cutting board with parchment.

2. For *Crust*, sift almond flour into medium mixing bowl. Add baking soda, vanilla and salt.

3. In a small mixing bowl, whisk eggs and date butter. Add flour mixture and mix to combine. Add oil, ghee or butter and mix until malleable dough comes together.

4. Roll in plastic wrap or wrap tightly in parchment and refrigerate for 15 minutes.

5. Heat medium pan over medium heat.

6. Chop strawberries and add to hot pan with honey, vanilla and salt. Cook strawberries down until juices thicken and reduce, about 10 minutes. Stir occasionally.

7. Remove dough from refrigerator. Roll out dough on parchment covered cutting board to about 1/8 inch thick rectangle with rolling pin. Use sharp knife or pizza cutter to cut dough into 4 rectangles.

8. Scoop equal portions of *Filling* into center of one side of each dough rectangle. Fold bare half of dough over filled half. Press edges together, letting any trapped air escape. Crimp edges of dough together with fork. Repeat with remaining dough.

9. Arrange pastries on prepared sheet pan and bake 15 - 20 minutes, or until golden and cooked through.

10. Remove from oven and serve immediately. Or allow to cool and serve room temperature.

11. Reheat in toaster, if preferred.

Orange Anzac Cookies

Prep Time: 5 minutes

Cook Time: 25 minutes

Servings: 12

INGREDIENTS

3/4 cup almond flour

3/4 cup sliced almonds

3/4 cup flaked or shredded coconut

1/4 cup date butter (raw honey or agave)

1/4 cup coconut oil (or ghee or cacao butter, melted)

1 orange (or tangerine or Clementine)

1/2 teaspoon baking soda

1/4 teaspoon ground ginger

INSTRUCTIONS

1. Preheat oven to 300 degrees F. Line sheet pan with parchment sheet or baking mat.

2. In medium mixing bowl, combine almond flour, sliced almonds and coconut.

3. Zest *then* juice orange into small mixings bowl. Add date butter and oil or melted butter. Mix to combine.

4. Add wet mixture to dry mixture and mix until dough comes together.

5. Form 12 large biscuits with tablespoon or scoop. Place on prepared sheet pan and flatten slightly.

6. Bake for 25 - 30 minutes, until golden. Remove from oven and let cool slightly before serving.
7. Serve warm. Or allow to cool completely and store in airtight container.

Cocoa Zucchini Muffin

Prep Time: 10 minutes

Cook Time: 15 minutes

Servings: 12

INGREDIENTS

1 1/2 cups almond flour

2 cage-free eggs

1 small zucchini (about 1 cup grated)

1/2 cup unsweetened applesauce

1/4 cup date butter (or agave or raw honey)

1/4 cup coconut oil (or cacao or coconut butter, melted)

1/4 cup cocoa powder

2 tablespoons ground chia seed (or flax meal)

1 teaspoon baking soda

1 teaspoon baking powder

1 teaspoon vanilla

1 teaspoon ground cinnamon

1 teaspoon ground black pepper

1/2 teaspoon Celtic sea salt

1/4 cup cocoa nibs or chocolate chips (optional)

INSTRUCTIONS

1. Preheat oven to 350 degrees F. Line muffin pan with paper liners or lightly coat with coconut oil.

2. Add eggs, oil or melted butter, applesauce and date butter to food processor or high-speed blender. Process until thick, light mixture forms, about 1 - 2 minutes.

3. Sift almond flour, cocoa powder, chia or flax meal, baking soda and powder, salt and spices into processor. Process to combine, about 1 minute.

4. Grate zucchini and stir in with cocoa nibs or chocolate chips (optional).

5. Use scoop or tablespoon to pour batter into prepared muffin pan. Bake for about 15 - 20 minutes, until toothpick inserted into center comes out clean.

6. Remove from oven and let cool about 5 minutes.

7. Serve warm. Or let cool completely and serve room temperature.

Crunchy Almond Butter Granola Bar

Prep Time: 30 minutes

Servings: 8

INGREDIENTS

1 1/2 cup raw almonds

1 cup crunchy almond butter

1/4 cup flax seed (or chia seed)

1/2 cup dried pitted dates

2/3 cup shredded or flaked coconut

1/3 cup raw pumpkin seeds

1/2 teaspoon ground cinnamon

1/2 teaspoon vanilla

1 teaspoon Celtic sea salt

INSTRUCTIONS

1. Line loaf pan with parchment paper.
2. Add flax or chia to food processor or high-speed blender and process until finely ground, about 1 - 2 minutes.
3. Add 1 cup almonds and process until thick, smooth paste forms, up to 5 minutes.
4. Add dates and process until thick, fairly smooth mixture forms about 1 - 2 minutes. Transfer to medium mixing bowl.
5. Add remaining 1/2 cup almonds, almond butter, coconut, pumpkin seeds, cinnamon, vanilla, and salt. Stir to combine with large wooden spoon.

6. Transfer mixture to parchment lined pan and firmly press into bottom with hands or spatula. Place in refrigerator for 20 minutes.

7. Remove from refrigerator and cut into bars.

8. Serve chilled. Or allow to warm to room temperature and serve.

Raw Island Sweet Bread

Prep Time: 10 minutes

Dehydrating Time: 6 - 8 hours

Servings: 8

INGREDIENTS

1 mango

1 guava

1/2 cup dried pineapple

1/2 cup flaked or shredded coconut

1 cup dried pitted dates

1/3 cup ground flax seed (or chia seed)

1 teaspoon ground ginger

1/4 teaspoon Celtic sea salt

INSTRUCTIONS

1. Cut mango in half around pit. Slice flesh in peel lengthwise and crosswise to create cubes, then invert peel and cut flesh from peel. Add mango to food processor or high-speed blender.
2. Cut guava and half and scoop out seeds, if preferred. Scoop flesh from rind and add to processor.
3. Add pineapple, coconut, dates, flax, ginger and salt to processor. Process until mixture is well ground and sticks together, about 2 minutes.
4. Line dehydrator tray with dehydrator or parchment sheet.

5. Form mixture into 2 loaves and place on lined dehydrator tray. Place in dehydrator and dehydrate at 115 degrees F for 2 hours. Reduce to 110 degrees F and dehydrate another 4 - 6 hours.

6. Remove from dehydrator and slice. Transfer to serving dish and serve immediately. Or store in airtight container.

Soft Baked Poppy Seed Pretzel

Prep Time: 15 minutes

Cook Time: 20 minutes

Servings: 4

INGREDIENTS

1 cup coconut flour

1/2 cup tapioca flour

1/2 cup coconut oil (or cacao or coconut butter)

1/2 cup water

1 cage-free egg

2 tablespoons apple cider vinegar

1/2 teaspoon baking soda

1/2 teaspoon baking powder

Topping

1 tablespoon coconut oil (or full-fat coconut milk)

1 - 2 tablespoons poppy seeds

INSTRUCTIONS

1. Preheat oven to 350 degrees F. Heat medium pan over medium-high heat. Line sheet pan with parchment or baking mat.

2. Add oil or butter, water, vinegar and salt to pot. Bring to a boil and remove from heat.

3. Whisk in tapioca flour. Stir until mixture congeals and comes together.

4. Stir in baking soda and baking powder. Continue mixing for a minute. Mixture will foam and expand. Let mixture sit and cool about 5 minutes.

5. Sift in coconut flour. Mix partially, then beat in egg. Blend until combined. Excess coconut flour may sit in bottom of bowl.

6. Turn out dough onto cutting board dusted with any excess coconut flour from mixture. Knead dough for 2 minutes.

7. Cut dough into 4 equal portions. Roll out pieces into ropes and twist to form classic pretzel twist. Pinch together any crumbled dough.

8. Arrange pretzels on lined sheet pan. For *Topping*, brush with coconut oil or milk and sprinkle generously with poppy seeds.

9. Place sheet pan in oven and bake about 25 minutes, until golden cooked through.

10. Serve warm. Or allow to cool and serve room temperature.

Superfood Granola

Prep Time: 5 minutes

Servings: 1

INGREDIENTS

1/2 cup raw almonds

1/3 cups raw walnuts

1/3 cups cashews

1/4 cup raw pumpkin seeds

1/4 cup shredded or flaked coconut

2 - 3 dried pitted dates

2 tablespoons pomegranate seeds (or goji or noni berries)

1/2 teaspoon Celtic sea salt

Pinch vanilla

Water

INSTRUCTIONS

1. Chop almonds, walnuts and dates by hand. Or add to clean food processor or high-speed blender and pulse to roughly chop.

2. Add to small bowl with pumpkin seeds, coconut, seeds or berries, and vanilla. Mix to combine.

3. Transfer to serving dish and serve immediately. Or store in airtight container.

Salt and Vinegar Dehydrated Kale Chips

Prep Time: 10 minutes

Dehydrating Time: 4 - 6 hours

Servings: 4

INGREDIENTS

2 kale heads (or 1.5 - 2 lbs kale leaves)

3 tablespoons coconut oil (or walnut, almond or sesame oil.)

1 tablespoon coconut aminos (or tamari or liquid aminos)

1 tablespoon coconut vinegar (or apple cider vinegar)

1 tablespoon Celtic sea salt

INSTRUCTIONS

1. Wash and spin dry kale. Remove tough spine and chop or tear into pieces.
2. Add kale pieces to large mixing bowl with oil, aminos, vinegar and salt and spices. Toss to coat.
3. Add single layer of coated kale to dehydrator tray and place in dehydrator. Dehydrate at 115 degrees F for 4 - 6 hours, depending on desired crispiness.
4. Remove kale from dehydrator and transfer to serving dish.
5. Serve immediately. Or store in airtight container.

Caribbean Jerked Beef Jerky

Prep Time: 10 minutes*

Dehydrating Time: 4 - 8 hours

Servings: 4

INGREDIENTS

4 oz (1/4 lb) grass-fed beef

2 tablespoons coconut aminos (or liquid aminos or tamari)

2 tablespoons lemon juice (or apple cider vinegar)

2 teaspoons raw honey (or agave or date butter)

1/4 teaspoon ground cloves

1/2 teaspoon ground cinnamon

1/2 teaspoon chipotle chile powder

3/4 teaspoon ground allspice

1 teaspoon dried thyme leaves

1 teaspoon ground black pepper

2 teaspoons cayenne pepper

2 teaspoons garlic powder

1 tablespoons Celtic sea salt

INSTRUCTIONS

1. Prepare two parchment sheets. Lay one on cutting board.
2. Cut slice beef into 1/4 inch strips and lay in single layer on parchment. Pound with tenderizing side of kitchen mallet. Cover beef with second parchment sheet, then pound with flat side of tenderizing mallet to 1/8 inch thickness.

3. *Place beef strips in medium mixing bowl or shallow dish. Add coconut aminos, lemon juice, salt and spices. Mix well to coat. Cover and place in refrigerator for 8 hours, or overnight.

4. Remove beef from refrigerator and lay in single layer on dehydrator trays. Place in dehydrator and dehydrate at 120 degrees F for 4 - 8 hours.

5. After 4 hours dehydrating time, remove trays from dehydrator and test beef by bending. If it cracks, remove and serve immediately. Or store in airtight container.

6. If still flexible, place back in dehydrator and continue dehydrating up to 4 hours, or until desired texture is achieved.

Fennel Seed Flax Crackers

Prep Time: 10 minutes

Dehydrating Time: 12 - 20 hours

Servings: 4

INGREDIENTS

Medium bunch fennel leaves

2 cups ground flax seed

2/3 cup whole flax seed

1 tablespoon fennel seeds

1 teaspoon Celtic sea salt

2 2/3 cups water

INSTRUCTIONS

1. Place parchment paper or dehydrator sheets on two dehydrator trays.
2. Finely mince fennel leaves. Add to large mixing bowl with seeds, salt and water. Mix until well combined.
3. Spread batter on prepared sheets. Place trays in dehydrator and set to 120 degrees F for 1 hour. Reduce temperature to 105 degrees F for remainder of dehydrating time.
4. After 4 hours dehydrating time, remove trays from dehydrator and use knife to score crackers in preferred shape and size. Place back in dehydrator and continue dehydrating another 4 hours.
5. Remove trays from dehydrator. Peel crackers from sheets and break apart along score lines. Place crackers directly on dehydrator

tray and continue dehydrating another 4 - 12 hours, depending on desired crispness.

6. Remove crackers from dehydrator and serve with your favorite raw dips, spreads and salsas. Or store in an airtight container up to 4 weeks.

Chocolate Nib Trail Mix

Prep Time: 5 minutes

Servings: 4

INGREDIENTS

1/2 cup raw almonds

1/2 cup raw pumpkin seeds

1/2 cup cashews

1/4 cup golden raisins

1/2 cup organic chocolate chips (or chocolate bark or cacao nibs)

INSTRUCTIONS

1. Roughly chop chocolate bark, if using. Add chocolate or cacao nibs to medium mixing bowl with raisins and nuts. Mix to combine.

2. Transfer to serving dish and serve immediately. Or store in cool dry place in airtight container.

Tart Cherry Lime Energy Bar

Prep Time: 25 minutes

Servings: 6

INGREDIENTS

1 cup dried tart cherries

1/4 cup dried pitted dates

1/3 cup warm water

1 lime

1 cup raw almonds

1/4 teaspoon ground ginger

1/4 teaspoon vanilla

1/8 teaspoon Celtic sea salt

INSTRUCTIONS

1. Zest and juice lime into small mixing bowl. Add warm water and dried cherries. Toss to coat and set aside 10 minutes.
2. Line loaf pan with parchment paper.
3. Add nuts and dates to food processor or high-speed blender. Drain soaked cherries and add to processor with cinnamon, vanilla and salt. Process for about 1 minute, until mixture is coarsely ground and sticks together when pressed.
4. Scrape mixture into prepared loaf pan and press firmly into bottom with hands or spatula.
5. Place in refrigerator and chill for 10 minutes. Remove and cut into 6 bars.
6. Serve immediately. Or store in refrigerator up to 2 weeks.

Blueberry Licorice Fruit Rolls

Prep Time: 15 minutes

Dehydrating Time: 6 hours

Servings: 6

INGREDIENTS

1 cup dried blueberries

1 cup blueberries (fresh or thawed)

1 teaspoon ground star anise

2 tablespoons ground chia or flax seed (optional)

Water (optional)

INSTRUCTIONS

1. Add fresh or thawed blueberries to food processor or high-speed blender and process until smooth, about 30 seconds.
2. Add dried blueberries and process until smooth, about 1 minute. Set aside 10 minutes.
3. Add anise and ground chia or flax (optional) to processor. Process with enough water to reach desired consistency. Mixture should be spreadable but not runny.
4. Line dehydrator tray with dehydrator or parchment sheet.
5. Spread mixture onto sheet 1/4 inch thick in large rectangle with spatula. Place in dehydrator and dehydrate on 115 degrees F for 4 hours.
6. Remove from dehydrator and use offset spatula to gently peel leather from sheet and flip over. Place back in dehydrator and dehydrate another 2 hours.

7. Remove from dehydrator and cut into strips. Or roll up and cut into logs. Transfer to serving dish and serve immediately.

Traditional Almond Macarons

Prep Time: 30 minutes

Cook Time: 15 minutes

Servings: 12

INGREDIENTS

2 large cage-free egg whites (room temperature)

1 cup almond flour

1/2 cup coconut sugar (or date butter, raw honey or agave)

1/2 teaspoon vanilla

INSTRUCTIONS

1. Preheat oven to 350 degrees F. Line sheet pan with parchment paper or baking mat.
2. Beat egg whites with hand mixer until white and frothy, about 2 minutes.
3. Add almond flour, sweetener and vanilla to food processor or high-speed blender. Process to combine, about 30 seconds.
4. Add egg whisked egg whites to processor and process until smooth paste forms, about 3 - 5 minutes.
5. Roll dough into small balls and place on prepared sheet pan. Flatten slightly with hand. Tap sheet pan on edge of counter to release any air bubbles, if preferred.
6. Bake for 10 - 15 minutes, until set and just golden.
7. Remove from oven and transfer full parchment sheet onto wire rack to cool completely. Do not try to remove warm cookies from parchment.

8. Allow to cool completely. Then peel from parchment and transfer to serving dish.

9. Serve room temperature.

Sweet Vanilla Shortbread Biscuits

Prep Time: 5 minutes

Cook Time: 20 minutes

Servings: 12

INGREDIENTS

1 2/3 cups almond flour

2/3 cup almonds (blanched, skinless)

1/4 cup coconut oil (or cacao butter or coconut butter, melted)

1/4 cup date butter (or raw honey or agave)

1 Madagascar whole vanilla bean

1/4 teaspoon baking soda

1/4 teaspoon Celtic sea salt (plus extra)

INSTRUCTIONS

1. Preheat oven to 300 degrees F. Line sheet pan with parchment or baking mat.
2. Add almonds to food processor or high-speed blender and process until finely ground, about 2 minutes.
3. Add ground almonds to medium mixing bowl. Sift in almond flour, baking soda and salt.
4. Split vanilla bean pod in half and scrap insides into small mixing bowl. Add oil or melted butter and date butter. Mix to combine.
5. Pour vanilla mixture into flour mixture and mix to form dough.
6. Use mini ice cream scoop or tablespoon to drop portions of dough onto prepared sheet pan. Bake for 20 minutes , or until lightly browned.

7. Remove from oven and let cool at least 5 minutes.

8. Serve warm. Or let cool completely and serve room temperature.

Cherry Fig Newton Cookies

Prep Time: 10 minutes

Cook Time: 15 minutes

Servings: 12

INSTRUCTIONS

Cookie Dough

1 1/2 cups almond flour

1/4 cup dried pitted dates

1/4 cup date butter (or agave or honey)

1/4 cup coconut oil (or cacao or coconut butter, melted)

1 teaspoon vanilla

1/4 teaspoon Celtic sea salt

Cherry Fig Filling

1/2 cup dried black mission figs

1/4 cup pitted cherries (fresh or thawed)

1/4 teaspoon ground ginger

INSTRUCTIONS

1. Preheat oven to 350 degrees F. Line sheet pan with parchment or baking mat.
2. For *Cookie Dough*, Add dried dates, date butter, and oil or melted butter to food processor or high-speed blender. Process until coarsely ground, about 1 - 2 minutes.
3. Sift almond flour and salt into medium mixing bowl. Add date mixture to flour mixture and mix to combine. Set aside.

4. For *Filling*, remove stems from figs and add to clean food processor or high-speed blender with cherries and ginger. Process until smooth mixture forms, about 2 minutes. Set aside.

5. Divide dough in half. Roll first half of dough into long, thin rectangle about 1/4 inch thick between 2 parchment sheets.

6. Spread 1/2 of *Cherry Fig Filling* along one side of the dough, long-ways.

7. Use parchment to fold dough in half along long edge so plain dough covers side with *Cherry Fig Filling*. Dough should resemble flattened log.

8. Press edges of dough together for tight seal. Place on prepared sheet pan. Repeat with remaining *Cookie Dough* and *Cherry Fig Filling*.

9. Bake for 12 - 15 minutes, or until the edges are golden brown.

10. Remove from the oven and let cool about 5 minutes. Then slice logs into 2 inch cookies.

11. Serve immediately. Or allow to cool completely and serve room temperature.

Lemon Coconut Pinwheels

Prep Time: 10 minutes

Cook Time: 20 minutes

Servings: 12

INGREDIENTS

Dough

2 cups almond flour

1 cage-free egg

2 tablespoon raw honey (or agave or date butter)

1 teaspoon vanilla

1/2 teaspoon baking powder

1/4 teaspoon Celtic sea salt

Filling

1/4 cup shredded or flaked coconut

1 lemon

2 tablespoons raw honey (or agave or date butter)

INSTRUCTIONS

1. Preheat oven to 300 degrees F. Line sheet pan with parchment or baking mat. Prepare 2 additional sheets of parchment.

2. For *Dough*, add flour, egg, honey, vanilla, baking powder and salt to medium mixing bowl. Blend with wooden spoon, then knead with hands to form thick dough, about 1 minute.

3. Divide dough in half. Place half of dough in small mixing bowl.

4. For *Filling*, add zest then juice lemon into small bowl. Add honey and coconut. Mix until well combined.

5. Roll out each half of dough separately on parchment sheets. Roll into equal rectangles.

6. Place *Filling* rectangle on top of plain dough. Use parchment to help roll dough tightly along long edge into log.

7. Use sharp knife to cut log into 1/4 thick round slices. Place cookies on prepared sheet pan. Bake for about 10 minutes, until edges are golden brown.

8. Remove from oven and let cool about 5 minutes.

9. Serve warm. Or let cool completely and serve room temperature.

Raisin Cinnamon Rugalach

Prep Time: 25 minutes

Cook Time: 20 minutes

Servings: 12

INSTRUCTIONS

Crust

2 cups almond flour

2 cage-free eggs

2 tablespoons coconut oil

2 tablespoons cacao butter (or or coconut butter or coconut cream)

2 tablespoons date butter (or raw honey or agave)

1 teaspoon baking powder

1/2 teaspoon baking soda

1/2 teaspoon vanilla

1/4 teaspoon ground cinnamon

1/4 teaspoon Celtic sea salt

Filling

2/3 cup California raisins

2/3 cup golden raisins

1/4 organic rum (or water)

2 tablespoons date butter (or raw honey or agave)

1/2 teaspoon vanilla

2 teaspoons ground cinnamon

INSTRUCTIONS

1. For *Crust*, sift almond flour into medium mixing bowl. Add baking soda and powder, vanilla, cinnamon and salt.

2. Whisk eggs and date butter in small mixing bowl, then add to flour mixture and combine. Slowly add coconut oil and butter or cream until malleable dough comes together.

3. Roll in plastic wrap or wrap tightly in parchment and refrigerate for 15 minutes.

4. Preheat oven to 350 degrees F. Line sheet pan with parchment or baking mat. Cover cutting board with parchment. Heat medium pan over medium-high heat.

5. For *Filling*, bring 1/4 cup rum or water to simmer In small pot. Add to small heat safe mixing bowl with raisins, vanilla and 1 teaspoon cinnamon. Mix well to combine and set aside about 5 minutes.

6. Remove dough from refrigerator. Roll dough out on parchment covered cutting board to about 1/8 inch thick rectangle with rolling pin.

7. Spread date butter over dough, then sprinkle on remaining 1 teaspoon cinnamon. Stir raisins in bowl again, then sprinkle over dough. Use sharp knife or pizza cutter to cut dough into 12 rectangles.

8. Roll up dough pieces and arrange on prepared sheet pan. Bake for 15 - 20 minutes, or until dough is golden brown and cooked through.

9. Remove from oven and allow to cool about 5 minutes.

10. Serve immediately. Or allow to cool completely and serve room temperature.

Cranberry Pistachio Biscotti

Prep Time: 15 minutes

Cook Time: 45 minutes*

Servings: 6

INGREDIENTS

1 cup almond flour

1/2 cup coconut flour

1/2 cup raw honey (or date butter or agave)

1/4 cup pistachios

1/4 cup dried cranberries

1/2 teaspoon vanilla

1/2 teaspoon baking soda

1/4 teaspoon Celtic sea salt

INSTRUCTIONS

1. Preheat oven to 350 degrees F. Line sheet pan with parchment paper. Heat medium pan over medium heat.

2. In medium mixing bowl, blend almond flour, coconut flour, baking soda and salt with hand mixer or whisk.

3. Beat in honey and vanilla until well combined and thick, sticky dough forms. Mix in pistachios and cranberries with wooden spoon.

4. Form dough into flattened, uniform mound about 1 inch thick on sheet pan. Pat down mound to keep any nuts from sticking out.

5. Bake for about 15 minutes. Remove from oven and allow to cool for about 15 minutes.

6. Use a very sharp serrated knife to carefully cut biscotti log into 1/2 - 2/3 inch slices. Hold on to the mound and cut on a diagonal. If it becomes crumbly, stick it back together.
7. Lay slices on their sides and return to oven for 15 minutes.
8. *Turn oven off and leave oven door open a crack. Allow biscotti to cool and dry for at least 2 hours.
9. Serve room temperature.

Double Chocolate Scone

Prep Time: 10 minutes

Cook Time: 25 minutes

Servings: 8

INGREDIENTS

2 cups almond flour

1/3 cup arrowroot flour

1 cage-free egg

1/4 cup coconut oil (or cacao or coconut butter, melted)

2 tablespoons raw honey (or agave)

2 tablespoons raw cocoa powder

2 teaspoons baking powder

1/2 teaspoon vanilla

1/2 teaspoon Celtic sea salt

1/2 cup organic chocolate chips (or chocolate bark or cacao nibs)

INSTRUCTIONS

1. Preheat oven to 350 degrees F. Line sheet pan with parchment or coat with coconut oil.

2. Whisk together almond flour, arrowroot flour, cocoa, baking powder, salt and vanilla in large mixing bowl.

3. In small mixing bowl, combine egg, and honey with hand mixer or whisk. Beat briskly while slowly pouring in oil or melted butter.

4. Add egg mixture to flour mixture blend and mix until well combined.

5. Roughly chop chocolate bark, if using. Fold in chocolate or cacao nibs until incorporated. Form dough into ball and place on sheet pan . Pat down to flatten to about 1/2 inch thick circle.

6. Cut into eight wedges with pizza cutter or sharp knife. Arrange at least 1 inch apart on prepared sheet pan.

7. Bake for 20 - 25 minutes , or until edges are browned.

8. Remove from oven and let cool completely.

9. Serve room temperature.

Sweet Almond Balls

Prep Time: 15 minutes

Servings: 12

INGREDIENTS

1/2 cup dried pitted dates

1/3 cup dried apricots

1/3 cup almonds (toasted or roasted, if preferred)

1/4 cup flaked or shredded coconut

1/2 tablespoon raw honey (or agave)

INSTRUCTIONS

1. Add apricots and dates to food processor or high-speed blender. Process until finely chopped, about 1 - 2 minutes.

2. Add almonds and coconut to processor. Process until well ground, about 2 minutes. Add honey and pulse until mixture sticks together, about 30 seconds.

3. Form mixture into 12 balls.

4. Serve immediately. Or store in airtight container in refrigerator up to 2 weeks.

Sesame Seed Date Balls

Prep Time: 15 minutes

Cook Time: 10 minutes

Servings: 12

INGREDIENTS

1 cup dried pitted dates

1/2 cup raw macadamia nuts (or almonds or cashews)

1/2 cup raw almonds (or hazelnuts or cashews)

2 oranges (about 1/2 cup juice)

2 tablespoons sesame seeds

1/4 teaspoon ground cinnamon

1/4 teaspoon ground ginger

INSTRUCTIONS

1. Juice oranges into small pot. Add dates and spices. Heat over medium heat and simmer about 10 minutes, until dates soften. Stir occasionally. Remove from heat and set aside about 5 minutes.

2. Heat small pan over medium heat. Add sesame seeds and toast until golden, about 5 minutes. Stir frequently and do not burn. Remove from heat and transfer to small dish.

3. Add nuts to food processor or high-speed blender. Process until finely chopped, about 1 - 2 minutes. Add cooled date mixture to nuts and process until mixture sticks together, about 1 minute.

4. Form date mixture into 12 - 18 balls and roll around in toasted sesame seeds to coat well.

5. Serve immediately. Or store in airtight container in refrigerator up to 2 weeks.

Salted Pretzel Rods

Prep Time: 15 minutes

Cook Time: 20 minutes

Servings: 12

INGREDIENTS

1 1/2 cups almond flour

3 tablespoons coconut flour

3 cage-free eggs

2 tablespoons ghee (or cacao butter or coconut oil, melted)

2 tablespoons Celtic sea salt

1 teaspoon water

INSTRUCTIONS

1. Beat 2 eggs in small mixing bowl with hand mixer to whisk. Set aside.

2. In medium bowl, sift almond flour, 1/2 teaspoon salt, and butter or oil. Mix to combine.

3. Add beaten eggs and 1 tablespoon coconut flour. Mix well. Let mixture sit 1 minute, then add second tablespoon of coconut flour. Blend again and let sit another minute. Add last tablespoon of coconut flour. Mix and set aside 5 minutes.

4. Preheat oven to 350 degrees F. Line sheet pan with parchment or baking mat.

5. Take portion of dough about the size of a golf ball and roll into long, thin log. Place on prepared sheet pan. Repeat with remaining dough.

6. Place pan in oven and bake 10 minutes.
7. Beat remaining egg in small bowl with 1 teaspoon water.
8. Remove pan from oven. Increase oven temperature to 400 degrees F.
9. Lightly brush tops of pretzels with the egg wash and sprinkle with generously with remaining salt.
10. Once oven is preheated, return pan to oven and bake 5 minutes.
11. Remove from oven and let cool slightly.
12. Serve warm. Or cool completely and serve room temperature.

Honey and Spice Nuts

Prep Time: 5 minutes

Cook Time: 5 minutes

Servings: 8

INGREDIENTS

1 cup almonds

1 cup walnuts

1 cup pecans

1 cup hazelnuts (or macadamia nuts)

1/4 cup raw honey (or agave or date butter)

1 teaspoon Celtic sea salt

1 teaspoon paprika (or smoked paprika or Hungarian paprika)

1/2 teaspoon chili powder

1/2 teaspoon ground cumin

1/2 teaspoon ground black pepper

1/2 teaspoon ground ginger

1/2 teaspoon ground cinnamon

1/4 teaspoon vanilla

1/4 teaspoon ground cardamom (optional)

1/4 teaspoon ground clove (optional)

INSTRUCTIONS

1. Heat large cast iron pan or skillet over medium-high heat.
2. Combine salt and spices in small mixing bowl.
3. Add nuts and honey to large mixing bowl and toss to coat. Sprinkle spice mixture over nuts and stir to coat well.

4. Add coated nuts to hot pan and sauté until caramelized, about 5 minutes. Stir continuously and do not burn.

5. Transfer nuts to sheet pan and spread in single layer to cool at least 5 minutes.

6. Transfer to serving dish and serve warm. Or cool completely and serve room temperature.

Pecan Pie Brittle

Prep Time: 15 minutes*

Cook Time: 10 minutes

Servings: 8

INGREDIENTS

1/2 - 1 cup raw pecans

1/2 cup honey raw honey (or agave)

1/2 cup date butter (or raw honey or agave)

1/2 cup coconut oil (or ghee or cacao butter, melted)

1/2 cup coconut cream concentrate (or coconut butter)

1/4 cup nut butter (for softer texture, if preferred)

2 teaspoons ground cinnamon

1 teaspoon vanilla

1/4 teaspoon Celtic sea salt

INSTRUCTIONS

1. Place medium pot over medium heat. Add 1 tablespoon oil or butter to hot pot.

2. Add your pecans to hot oiled pan. Stir frequently with heat-resistant spoon or spatula to toast, about 3 - 5 minutes. Do not burn.

3. Add sweeteners and mix well. Once hot and slightly thickened, add remaining oil or butter, coconut cream or butter, and nut butter (optional). Stir continuously to prevent burning.

4. Stir in cinnamon, vanilla and salt. Reduce heat to low and let simmer for 3 - 4 minutes.

5. Line square glass baking dish with parchment paper. Or place silicon baking dish over half-sheet pan.

6. Carefully pour hot mixture into prepared baking dish. Use spoon to spread pecans evenly throughout mixture.

7. Cover well with parchment, if preferred, and set aside in freezer at least 1 hour.

8. Remove from freezer and baking dish. Peel away parchment, if using. Crack brittle with kitchen mallet to break into pieces. Or score with knife and break into pieces by hand.

9. Serve immediately. Or allow to warm and serve room temperature

Meat Cookbook

All-Natural Chicken Sausage

Prep Time: 5 minutes

Cook Time: 10 minutes

Servings: 4

INGREDIENTS

20 oz (1 1/4 lb) chicken (ground meat or whole pieces)

1/2 teaspoon all spice

1 teaspoon fennel seed

1 teaspoon ground sage

1 teaspoon dried thyme

1 teaspoon ground black pepper

1 teaspoon Celtic sea salt

Natural or synthetic sausage casing (optional)

Piping or kitchen bag (optional)

Coconut oil (for cooking)

INSTRUCTIONS

1. Heat medium skillet over medium heat and lightly coat with coconut oil.

2. Remove chicken skin and bones from pieces and coarsely grind in food processor, high-speed blender or meat grinder, if using.

3. Add ground chicken to medium mixing bowl with salt and spices and mix well.

4. Use meat grinder to stuff mixture into casing. Or scoop mixture into piping bag with no tip or kitchen bag with 1 inch corner cut

off, and pipe into casing. Twist casing tightly in opposite directions to section off 4-inch links while stuffing.

5.   Or form into 8 - 12 round patties with hands.

6. Place links or patties in hot oiled skillet. Cook links about 4 - 5 minutes per side, until golden brown and cooked through. Or cook patties about 3 - 4 minutes per side, until golden brown and crisp. Turn halfway through cooking.

7. Drain cooked sausage on paper towel. Serve hot.

Gourmet Turkey Legs

Prep Time: 10 minutes*

Cook Time: 1 hour 20 minutes

Servings: 4

INGREDIENTS

2 large turkey legs

1/2 teaspoon garlic powder

1/2 teaspoon onion powder

1/2 teaspoon dried rosemary

1/2 teaspoon dried thyme

1/2 paprika (or smoked paprika or Hungarian paprika)

1/2 teaspoon Celtic sea salt

1/2 teaspoon ground black pepper

1 1/2 tablespoon coconut oil

Brine

4 cups water

1/4 cup Celtic sea salt

1/4 cup raw honey (or agave or date butter)

INSTRUCTIONS

1. *For *Brine*, add water, salt and sweetener to wide, shallow container. Mix to combine. Add turkey legs and submerge completely in *Brine*. Marinate in refrigerator 12 - 24 hours.

2. Preheat oven to 350 degrees F. Place wire rack over sheet pan.

3. Remove turkey legs from brine. Rub salt, spices and oil over turkey legs, and under skin.

4. Place coated turkey legs on wire rack and bake about 35 - 40 minutes. Carefully turn turkey legs over and bake another 35 - 40 minutes, until skin is crisp and meat is cooked through.

5. Remove from oven and let rest about 2 minutes. Then serve hot.

Classic Rack of Lamb with Mint Sauce

Prep Time: 5 minutes*

Cook Time: 25 minutes

Servings: 2

INGREDIENTS

1 rack of lamb with 7 - 8 ribs (about 3/4 lb)

2 tablespoons date butter (or raw honey or agave)

1 teaspoon fresh thyme

1 teaspoon fresh rosemary

1/2 teaspoon cracked black pepper (or ground black pepper)

1/2 teaspoon ground cinnamon (optional)

1 tablespoon coconut oil

Fresh Mint Sauce

1/2 cup fresh mint leaves

2 tablespoons raw honey (or agave or date butter)

1/3 cup apple cider vinegar or (coconut aminos)

INSTRUCTIONS

1. *Chop rosemary and thyme. Rub herbs, spices and salt into lamb. Cover and set aside 45 - 60 minutes.

2. Preheat oven to 475 degrees F. Coat baking dish just large enough to fit rack of lamb with coconut oil.

3. Place lamb in prepared baking dish and roast for 10 minutes. Reduce temperature to 375 degrees F and continue to cook for 10 - 15 minutes, for rare to medium-rare.

4. For *Fresh Mint Sauce*, add mint, vinegar and sweetener to food processor or high-speed blender. Process until smooth, about 1 - 2 minutes. Transfer to serving dish.

5. Remove lamb from oven and let rest about 5 minutes.

6. Cut rack of lamb into individual lamb chops and transfer to serving dish. Serve warm with *Fresh Mint Sauce*.

Modern Beef Haggis

Prep Time: 10 minutes

Cook Time: 3 hours

Servings: 4

INGREDIENTS

8 oz (1/2 lb) ground beef (or bison, elk, etc.)

8 oz (1/2 lb) lamb shoulder

4 oz (1/4 lb) calves liver

2 onions (yellow or white)

1/2 head cauliflower (about 1 cup riced)

1 cup beef stock

2 garlic cloves

1/2 teaspoon ground nutmeg

1/4 teaspoon ground coriander

1/2 teaspoon Celtic sea salt

1/2 ground white pepper (or ground black pepper)

1/4 cup ghee (or coconut oil or cacao butter)

Water

INSTRUCTIONS

1. Preheat oven to 300 degrees F. Generously coat baking dish with ghee, oil or butter.

2. Add liver to small pan with enough water to cover over high heat. Bring to simmer and cook about 5 minutes. Drain and set aside to cool.

3. Roughly chop cauliflower. Peel and roughly chop onions and garlic. Add to food processor with lamb shoulder and par-cooked liver. Process until coarsely ground, about 2 minutes.

4. Add ground beef, stock, salt, and spices and pulse to combine. Transfer to prepared baking dish and cover tightly with aluminum foil.

5. Place covered dish in roasting pan. Add water to roasting pan 3/4 of the way up side of baking dish.

6. Bake for 3 hours. Remove from oven and carefully remove foil. Let rest about 10 minutes.

7. Remove baking dish from roasting pan. To plate, place serving dish over baking dish and carefully invert. Slice haggis into wedges and serve hot with mashed parsnips or yams.

Bacon Filet Mignon Steak

Prep Time: 5 minutes

Cook Time: 20 minutes

Servings: 2

INGREDIENTS

2 (6 oz each) filet mignon steaks

2 thick slices nitrate-free bacon

Ground black pepper, to taste

Celtic sea salt, to taste

1 tablespoon coconut oil (optional)

Toothpicks

INSTRUCTIONS

1. Preheat oven to 350 degrees F. Heat medium oven-safe pan or skillet over medium heat.

2. Add bacon to hot pan. Cook and render out fat for about 5 minutes, until about halfway cooked. Remove bacon from pan and set aside, reserving bacon fat in pan. Add coconut oil to pan, if desired.

3. Wrap par-cooked bacon around steaks and secure with toothpick. Sprinkle steaks with salt and pepper to taste.

4. Add wrapped seasoned steaks to hot oiled pan and sear 2 minutes per side. Carefully flip half way through cooking.

5. Remove pan from stove and place in preheated oven. Cook about 8 - 10 minutes, until bacon is cooked through and steak is medium-rare.

6. Remove steaks from oven and transfer to cutting board. Set aside and let rest at least 2 minutes.
7. Transfer to serving dish and serve hot.

Beef Braciole with Tomato Sauce

Prep Time: 10 minutes

Cook Time: 1 hour 45 minutes

Servings: 6

INGREDIENTS

24 oz (1 1/2 lb) beef flank steak

2/3 cup coarse almond meal

2/3 cup nutritional yeast

1 garlic clove

Small bunch fresh Italian parsley

1 cup dry white wine (or apple cider)

2 teaspoons dried oregano

1 teaspoon garlic powder

1 teaspoon ground black pepper

1 teaspoon Celtic sea salt

3 (5 oz) cans organic tomato sauce

1/4 cup coconut oil

INSTRUCTIONS

1. Preheat oven to 350 degrees F. Heat oven-proof skillet over medium heat. Add 2 tablespoon coconut oil in hot pan.

2. Chop parsley. Peel and mince garlic. Add to medium mixing bowl with almond meal, nutritional yeast, 1 teaspoon dried oregano, 1/2 teaspoon salt and pepper, and 2 tablespoons coconut oil. Mix to combine.

3. Evenly coat flank steak with almond meal mixture. Roll up lengthwise and secure with kitchen twine. Season with remaining salt and pepper.

4. Place rolled steak in hot oiled pan. Brown about 2 minutes on each side. Add wine or cider and bring to simmer. Add tomato sauce, garlic powder and remaining oregano. Stir to combine.

5. Cover loosely with foil and bake for 1 hour, basting with the sauce every 30 minutes. Then carefully remove foil and bake another 30 minutes.

6. Carefully remove beef from sauce and remove twine. Cut into 1/2 inch slices and transfer to serving dish. Spoons sauce over beef and serve hot.

Roasted Stuffed Game Hen

Prep Time: 10 minutes

Cook Time: 75 minutes

Servings: 8

INGREDIENTS

2 (2 lbs each) whole Cornish game hens

4 large celery stalks (about 1/2 lb)

4 slices nitrate-free bacon

1 small red onion

1/2 cup chopped pecans

2 tablespoons dried thyme

2 teaspoons mustard powder

1 teaspoon paprika

1 teaspoon ground white pepper (or ground black pepper)

1 teaspoon Celtic Sea salt

2 tablespoons ghee (or coconut oil)

Apricot Jam

1/4 cup dried apricots

Water

INSTRUCTIONS

1. Preheat oven to 350 degrees F.
2. Rinse and remove entrails from game hens. Pat dry with paper towel. Set aside in oven-safe dish large enough to fit both birds with a little extra space. Use lidded dish if preferred.

3. Add spices to small mixing bowl and mix to combine. Rub spice mixture over hens, and beneath skin where possible.

4. Peel onion and chop. Chop celery and bacon. Add to medium mixing bowl with pecans and mix to combine.

5. Stuff hens with bacon mixture and lay in dish breast-side up. Add leftover stuffing mixture around hens in dish. Rub hens with ghee or coconut oil and add 1/2 inch of water to dish.

6. Cover dish with lid or aluminum foil and cook for 45 minutes. Remove dish from oven and carefully remove lid or foil. Place back in oven and cook for 30 minutes.

7. For *Apricot Jam*, add apricots to food processor or high-speed blender and process about 1 minute. Add enough water to reach thick, smooth consistency. Transfer to serving dish.

8. Remove game hens from oven and let rest about 5 - 10 minutes.

9. Carve hens and serve hot with stuffing and *Apricot Jam*.

BLT Burger Wrap

Prep Time: 5 minutes

Cook Time: 25 minutes

Servings: 6

INGREDIENTS

24 oz (1.5 lbs) ground turkey

18 slices nitrate-free bacon

2 medium tomatoes

6 large romaine lettuce leaves

1/2 teaspoon paprika (or smoked or Hungarian paprika)

1/2 teaspoon ground black pepper

1 teaspoon Celtic sea salt

INSTRUCTIONS

1. Heat large pan or skillet over medium heat.

2. Add bacon to hot pan or skillet. Cook about 5 - 6 minutes on each side, until browned and crisp. Flip halfway through cooking. Set aside on paper towel to drain. Reserve 4 tablespoons bacon fat in pan. Reserve remaining bacon fat for later use.

3. Add ground turkey, 1 tablespoon bacon fat, salt and spices to medium mixing bowl. Mix well with hands or large wooden spoon.

4. Form turkey mixture into 6 patties and add to hot oiled pan. Cook about 4 - 5 minutes on each side, for medium doneness. Flip halfway through cooking.

5. Remove burgers from pan and drain on paper towels.

6. Slice tomatoes. Lay lettuce leaves flat. Place burger patties on one end of lettuce and top with bacon and tomato slices. Wrap up burger in lettuce. Repeat with remaining burgers, bacon and veggies.
7. Transfer to serving dish and serve immediately.

Baked Pork Chops with Cinnamon Apples

Prep Time: 10 minutes

Cook Time: 30 minutes

Servings: 4

INGREDIENTS

Pork Chops

4 pork chops (bone-in or boneless)

1/2 cup almond flour

2 tablespoons coconut oil (or cacao butter or ghee)

1 sprig fresh rosemary

1 teaspoon dried thyme

Ground black pepper, to taste

Celtic sea salt, to taste

Coconut oil (for cooking)

Cinnamon Apples

4 tart apples

1/4 cup raw honey (or agave or date butter)

1 tablespoon ground cinnamon

2 tablespoons coconut oil (or cacao butter or ghee)

INSTRUCTIONS

1. Preheat oven to 350 degrees F. Heat large pan over medium heat. Add 2 tablespoons oil, butter or ghee to hot pan.

2. Lightly coat wire rack or slotted broiler pan with coconut oil. Place over sheet pan layered with aluminum foil to catch drippings.

3. For *Pork Chops*, pat pork chops dry and sprinkle with salt and pepper. Place on wire rack or broiler pan.

4. Remove rosemary needles from stem and chop. Add to small mixing bowl with almond flour, coconut oil, thyme, salt and pepper. Mix to form paste.

5. Press seasoned paste into top of each pork chop with fingers to form a 1/8 inch thick crust.

6. Place pork chops in oven and bake about 20 - 25 minutes.

7. For *Cinnamon Apples*, peel and core apple. Cut apples into thick slices and add to large mixing bowl with sweetener and cinnamon. Mix to combine.

8. Add seasoned apples to hot oiled pan. Sauté about 5 minutes, until aromatic and lightly browned. Reduce heat to medium-low and add 1/2 cup water.

9. Cover pan with lid or aluminum foil and simmer about 20 minutes, or until apples are tender. Stir occasionally.

10. Set oven to BROIL and move pork chops about 6 inches away from the heating element. Broil for about 5 minutes, until topping is browned. Rotate halfway through broiling, if necessary. Do not burn topping.

11. Transfer *Cinnamon Apples* to serving dish. Remove pork chops from oven and place over *Cinnamon Apples*.

12. Serve immediately.

Veal Scallopini with White Wine Sauce

Prep Time: 5 minutes

Cook Time: 10 minutes

Servings: 4

INGREDIENTS

16 oz (1 lb) veal cutlets

1/4 cup white wine (or apple cider)

1/2 large lemon

2 tablespoons capers

3 tablespoons bacon fat (or ghee)

1 tablespoon coconut oil

Celtic sea salt, to taste

Coconut oil (for cooking)

INSTRUCTIONS

1. Heat large pan over medium heat. Add 1 tablespoon coconut oil to hot pan.

2. Use kitchen mallet to pound cutlets into 1/4 inch thickness. Sprinkle with sea salt to taste.

3. Add veal to hot oiled pan and brown for 2 minutes on each side. Flip halfway through cooking. Remove veal from pan and transfer to serving dish.

4. Add capers to pan and sauté about 30 seconds. Add wine and reduce by half, about 2 minutes. Juice lemon into pan, and add bacon fat or ghee. Swirl or whisk to emulsify sauce.

5. Drizzle sauce over veal and serve warm.

Simple enison Stir-Fry

Prep Time: 5 minutes*

Cook Time: 10 minutes

Servings: 4

INGREDIENTS

16 oz (1 lb) venison

1 bell pepper (red, yellow or green)

1 small onion (white, red or yellow)

1 small carrot

1/3 cup button mushrooms (about 4 - 5)

2 tablespoons tamari (or coconut aminos or apple cider vinegar)

1 teaspoon raw honey (or agave or date butter)

1 garlic clove

1/2 inch piece fresh ginger

1/4 teaspoon allspice (optional)

1/2 teaspoon red pepper flakes

1 teaspoon ground black pepper

1 1/2 teaspoons Celtic sea salt

3 tablespoons bacon fat (or coconut oil)

INSTRUCTIONS

1. *Peel and mince garlic. Cut venison into 1/2 inch strips. Add to medium mixing bowl with 1 tablespoon bacon fat or coconut oil, and 1/2 of salt and spices. Mix to combine. Set aside in refrigerator at least 30 minutes.

2. Heat large pan or skillet over medium heat. Add 1 tablespoon bacon fat or coconut oil to hot pan.

3. Remove stem, seeds and veins from bell pepper. Peel onion. Slice pepper, onion, carrot and mushrooms. Peel and mince or grate ginger. Add to medium mixing bowl with remaining salt and spices.

4. Add seasoned veggies to hot oiled pan. Sauté until tender and lightly browned, about 2 minutes.

5. Add remaining bacon fat and or coconut oil, tamari and honey to pan. Add marinated venison and sauté until just cooked, about 2 - 3 minutes.

6. Transfer to serving dish and serve hot.

Bison Bacon Burger

Prep Time: 5 minutes

Cook Time: 25 minutes

Servings: 6

INGREDIENTS

24 oz (1.5 lbs) ground buffalo (or bison)

12 slices nitrate-free bacon

Celtic sea salt, to taste

Ground black pepper, to taste

Stone ground mustard (optional)

Burger Buns

1/4 cup almond flour

1/4 cup coconut flour

4 cage-free eggs

2 tablespoons coconut oil (or cacao butter or ghee, melted)

2 tablespoons unsweetened applesauce

1 teaspoon flax meal (or ground chia seed)

1 teaspoon baking powder

1/2 teaspoon Celtic sea salt

INSTRUCTIONS

1. Preheat oven to 350 degrees F. Heat large pan or skillet over medium heat. Line sheet pan with parchment paper, or lightly coat with coconut oil. Or lightly coat 6 mini round cake pans with coconut oil.

2. For *Burger Buns*, beat eggs, oil or butter, and applesauce in medium mixing bowl with hand mixer or whisk.

3. In large mixing bowl, sift together coconut flour, almond flour, flax or chia meal, baking powder and salt. Pour egg mixture into flour mixture and mix until combined.

4. Scoop thick batter onto prepared sheet pan in 6 rounds. Or pour into 6 prepared mini cake pans. Smooth batter with knife or spatula.

5. Place in oven and bake for 12 - 15 minutes, or until tops are firm to the touch and golden.

6. Add bacon to hot pan or skillet. Cook about 5 minutes on each side, until browned and crisp. Flip halfway through cooking. Set aside on paper towel to drain. Reserve bacon fat in pan.

7. Form ground buffalo into 6 patties. Sprinkle with salt and pepper to taste.

8. Add patties to hot oiled pan and cook about 4 - 5 minutes on each side, for medium doneness. Flip halfway through cooking.

9. Remove *Burger Buns* from oven and let cool at least 5 minutes.

10. Slice *Burger Buns* in half. Cut bacon in half and lay 2 pieces on each bottom bun. Top with a burger patty, and add another 2 pieces of bacon. Smear top bun with coarse-grain mustard (optional), and add top bun.

11. Transfer to serving dish and serve immediately.

Amazing Bacon Dog with Rémoulade

Prep Time: 10 minutes

Cook Time: 15 minutes

Servings: 4

INGREDIENTS

8 slices nitrate-free bacon

8 all-natural hot dog links (beef, pork, chicken, turkey, etc.)

Rémoulade

1/2 cup coconut cream (settled from full-fat canned coconut milk)

1/4 cup roasted red peppers

2 tablespoons spicy mustard (fine or coarse grain)

2 tablespoons organic tomato paste

1 small green onion (scallion)

1/2 teaspoon tamari (or coconut aminos or apple cider vinegar)

1 teaspoon smoked paprika (or paprika or Hungarian paprika)

1/4 teaspoon dried parsley

1/4 teaspoon Celtic sea salt

Pinch all spice (optional)

Pinch cayenne pepper (optional)

Toothpicks (optional)

INSTRUCTIONS

1. Preheat oven to 400 degrees F. Line sheet pan with parchment paper or aluminum foil, or wire rack.

2. Tightly wrap bacon around hot dogs. Secure bacon with toothpicks (optional). Place wrapped hot dogs on prepared sheet pan.

3. Bake 12 - 15 minutes, until bacon is cooked through and hot dogs are browned.

4. For *Rémoulade*, add coconut cream, roasted red peppers, mustard, tomato paste, green onion, tamari, salt and spices to food processor or high-speed blender. Process until smooth and creamy, about 1 minute. Transfer to serving dish.

5. Remove hot dogs from oven and transfer to serving dish. Serve hot with *Rémoulade*.

Pork Tenderloin with Apricot Sauce

Prep Time: 10 minutes*

Cook Time: 15 minutes

Servings: 4

INGREDIENTS

1 pork tenderloin

1 teaspoon dried rosemary

1 teaspoon dried thyme

1 teaspoon dried oregano

1 teaspoon dried basil

1 teaspoon dried marjoram (optional)

1/2 teaspoon ground black pepper

1 teaspoon Celtic sea salt

Apricot Sauce

1 cup dried apricots

2/3 cup water

1 teaspoon apple cider vinegar (or dry white wine)

INSTRUCTIONS

1. Preheat oven to 425 degrees F. Heat small pan over medium heat.

2. Rub tenderloin with salt and spices, then press into meat so it adheres. Place on sheet pan, or wire rack over sheet pan.

3. Roast for 10 - 15 minutes, until just cooked through and no pink remains. Remove pork from oven and let rest 10 minutes.

4. For *Apricot Sauce,* add dried apricots, water and vinegar to food processor or high-speed blender. Process until smooth, about 1 - 2 minutes.

5. Add *Apricot Sauce* to hot pan and reduce until slightly thickened. Stir well and do not let burn. Remove from heat.

6. Slice pork and transfer to serving dish. Top pork with *Apricot Sauce* and serve warm.

Gourmet Chicken Liver Pâté

Prep Time: 10 minutes*

Cook Time: 15 minutes

Servings: 6

INGREDIENTS

16 oz (1 lb) fresh chicken livers

1 cup kefir (or coconut milk)

1/2 cup coconut oil (or cacao butter or ghee)

1/4 cup red wine (or apple cider)

1 small-medium yellow onion

2 garlic cloves

2 tablespoons green peppercorns (jarred)

2 bay leaves

2 sprigs fresh thyme leaves

1/2 teaspoon Celtic sea salt

1/2 teaspoon ground black pepper

Chopped parsley leaves (optional garnish)

INSTRUCTIONS

1. *Clean livers well, then add to medium mixing bowl with kefir or coconut milk. Set aside for 2 hours. Then drain well.

2. Heat large pan or skillet over medium heat. Add 4 tablespoons oil or butter to pan.

3. Peel and chop onions and garlic. Add to hot pan and sauté until soft and fragrant, about 4 minutes.

4. Add chicken livers, 1 tablespoon drained peppercorns, bay leaves, thyme leaves, salt and pepper. Sauté until livers are lightly browned, about 5 minutes.

5. Add wine or cider and cook until most liquid is evaporated and livers are just cooked through and tender, about 5 minutes.

6. Remove from heat and let cool slightly. Remove and discard bay leaves.

7. Add liver mixture and remaining oil or butter to food processor or high-speed blender. Stir in the remaining peppercorns.

8. *Use spoon to pack mixture into 4 - 6 ceramic ramekins or molds. Cover with plastic wrap and refrigerate at least 6 hours, until firm.

9. Remove from refrigerator and serve with parsley (optional garnish).

Crispy Pan Seared Duck

Prep Time: 10 minutes

Cook Time: 15 minutes

Servings: 2

INGREDIENTS

2 (8 oz each) boneless duck breast halves (with skin and fat)

1 teaspoon raw honey

2 teaspoons dried thyme

1 sprig rosemary

1/2 teaspoon ground black pepper

1 teaspoons Celtic sea salt

INSTRUCTIONS

1. Heat medium pan or skillet over medium-high heat.
2. Rinse duck breast and pat dry with paper towel.
3. Rub rosemary spring between palms, then remove needles from stem and chop. Rub rosemary, thyme, salt and pepper into both sides of duck breasts.
4. Drizzle honey over fatty side of duck breast, then place in hot oiled pan, skin and fat side down. Let brown undisturbed for 5 minutes. Turn duck over with tongs and cook until desired doneness, 5 - 10 minutes for medium to well done.
5. Transfer duck breasts to cutting board and cover with aluminum foil. Set aside to rest 5 minutes.
6. Cut each duck breast in 1/2 inch diagonal slices. Transfer to serving dish and serve warm.

Cajun Spice Broiled Gator Tail

Prep Time: 10 minutes

Cook Time: 30 minutes

Servings: 4

INGREDIENTS

16 oz (1 lb) gator tail

1/2 teaspoon cayenne pepper

1 teaspoon garlic powder

1 teaspoon dried thyme

2 tablespoons paprika

1 tablespoon ground oregano

1 tablespoon ground white pepper (or ground black pepper)

1 tablespoon Celtic sea salt

Coconut oil (optional)

INSTRUCTIONS

1. Set oven to BROIL. Lightly coat sheet pan or skillet with coconut oil. Or place wire rack over sheet pan.

2. Cut gator meat into 1 inch cubes and add to medium mixing bowl. Add salt and spices and toss to coat.

3. Place on rack, sheet pan or skillet. Place in oven about 6 - 8 inches away from broiler and cook for 4 - 6 minutes, until meat is white and firm to the touch.

4. Remove from oven and transfer to serving dish. Serve hot.

Veggie Medley Stuffed Peppers

Prep Time: 10 minutes

Cook Time: 50 minutes

Servings: 4

INGREDIENTS

4 bell peppers

16 oz (1 lb) ground meat (beef, pork, chicken, turkey, etc.)

1/2 head cauliflower (1 cup riced)

1/2 cup roasted red peppers

1/4 cup sundried tomatoes

1/4 cup pecans

1/2 small onion (white, yellow or red)

2 tablespoons coconut oil

2 garlic cloves

Medium bunch fresh herbs (parsley, oregano, thyme, etc.)

1/4 teaspoon red pepper flakes

1 teaspoon ground white pepper (or black pepper)

1 teaspoon Celtic sea salt

Water

INSTRUCTIONS

1. Preheat oven to 350 degrees F.
2. Cut tops off peppers, then remove stems from tops and seeds and veins from bottoms of peppers. Leave bottoms of peppers hollow but do not pierce. Place in baking dish just large enough to fit peppers snuggly. Set aside.

3. Peel onion and garlic. Roughly chop onions, garlic and cauliflower. Add to food processor or high-speed blender with pecans. Pulse about 15 seconds.

4. Add tops of peppers, roasted red peppers, sundried tomatoes, ground meat, salt, pepper, and fresh herbs to processor. Process until coarsely ground, about 1 - 2 minutes.

5. Use large spoon to stuff peppers with mixture. Add 1/2 cup water to bottom of baking dish. Cover peppers with aluminum foil.

6. Bake 30 minutes. Carefully remove foil and continue baking uncovered 10 - 20 minutes, until stuffing is golden brown and cooked through .

7. Carefully remove from oven and transfer peppers to serving dish. Serve hot.

Walnut Sausage Stuffed Tomatoes

Prep Time: 10 minutes

Cook Time: 40 minutes

Servings: 4

INGREDIENTS

8 small-medium tomatoes (red, yellow, green, or any combination)

16 oz (1 lb) Italian sausage (sweet or spicy)

1 celery stalk

1/2 onion (white or yellow)

1/2 cup red radishes (about 6)

1/2 cup walnuts (or pecans, almonds, etc.)

1/3 cup nutritional yeast (optional)

6 large basil leaves basil

1 tablespoon fresh thyme leaves

Celtic sea salt, to taste

Ground black pepper, to taste

2 tablespoons bacon fat (or coconut oil)

INSTRUCTIONS

1. Preheat oven to 350 degrees F.
2. Cut tops off tomatoes, then remove stems from tops and seeds and juices from bottoms of tomatoes. Leave bottoms of tomatoes hollow but do not pierce. Place in baking dish just large enough to fit tomatoes snuggly. Set aside.
3. Peel onion and garlic. Mince or coarsely grate garlic, onion and radish. Finely dice celery and tops of tomatoes. Finely chop basil

and thyme leaves. Coarsely chop pecans. Add to medium mixing bowl with sausage, salt and pepper to taste, and nutritional yeast (optional). Mix well.

4. Use large spoon to stuff tomatoes with mixture. Drizzle bacon fat or coconut oil over tomatoes. Cover tomatoes with aluminum foil.

5. Bake 25 minutes. Carefully remove foil and continue baking uncovered 10 - 15 minutes, until stuffing is golden brown .

6. Carefully remove from oven and serve hot.

Sautéed Frog Legs with Lemon Butter Sauce

Prep Time: 10 minutes*

Cook Time: 15 minutes

Servings: 4

INGREDIENTS

12 pairs frog legs (fresh or thawed)

1 1/2 cups kefir (or coconut milk)

1/2 cup ghee (or cacao butter or coconut oil)

1 cup almond flour

2 garlic cloves

1/2 lemon

Small bunch fresh parsley

Ground black pepper, to taste (ground white pepper)

Celtic sea salt, to taste

INSTRUCTIONS

1. Separate each pair of frog legs with knife or kitchen shears. Add to medium mixing bowl with kefir. Set aside in refrigerator for 30 minutes.

2. Heat large pan or skillet over high heat. Add 1/4 cup ghee, butter or oil to hot pan.

3. Drain frog legs and pat dry with paper towels. Season to taste with salt and pepper.

4. Add almond flower to shallow dish. Add frog legs to almond flower, coat well, then shake off excess.

5. Add coated frog legs to hot oiled pan and cook 2 minutes on each side. Flip halfway through cooking. Remove frog legs from pan and transfer to serving dish.

6. Drain pan an carefully wipe with paper towel until clean. Add pan back to heat.

7. Peel garlic and finely chop. Add to hot pan with 1/4 cup ghee, butter or oil. Sauté and stir continuously about 1 minute, until garlic is fragrant.

8. Remove from heat and add squeeze of lemon juice, and salt and pepper to taste. Drizzle pan sauce over frog legs. Finely chop parsley and garnish.

9. Serve warm.

Healthy Gyro

Prep Time: 10 minutes

Cook Time: 30 minutes

Servings: 2

INGREDIENTS

2 large romaine lettuce leaves

1 tomato

1/2 small red onion

Gyro Meat

8 oz (1/2 lb) ground lamb

8 oz (1/2 lb) ground beef

1 small onion (white or yellow)

2 garlic cloves

1 teaspoon dried marjoram

1 teaspoon dried oregano

1 teaspoon dried rosemary

1 teaspoon ground black pepper

1 teaspoon Celtic sea salt

Coconut oil (for cooking)

Coconut Cream Tzatziki

1/2 small cucumber

1/4 cup coconut cream (settled from full-fat canned coconut milk)

1 teaspoon lemon juice

1/2 teaspoon apple cider vinegar

2 mint leaves

1 sprig fresh dill

1 garlic clove

1/4 teaspoon Celtic sea salt

INSTRUCTIONS

1. Preheat oven to 325 degrees F. Line small loaf pan with parchment or aluminum foil.

2. For *Gyro Meat*, peel white or yellow onion and add to food processor or high-speed blender. Process until finely ground, about 30 seconds. Turn out onto cheesecloth or paper towels. Squeeze or compress onions to remove as much liquid as possible.

3. Add drained onions back to processor. Peel garlic and add to processor with lamb, beef, herbs, salt and pepper. Process until mixture is smooth, about 2 - 3 minutes. Scrape down sides of bowl as necessary.

4. Add mixture to prepared loaf pan. Pack tightly and smooth top. Bake for 30 minutes. Remove from oven and allow to rest about 5 minutes.

5. For *Coconut Cream Tzatziki*, peel, seed and shred, grate or dice cucumber. Peel and mince garlic. Mince mint and dill. Add to small mixing bowl with coconut cream, lemon juice, salt and vinegar. Mix well, then set aside to chill in refrigerator.

6. Heat medium skillet over medium-high heat and lightly coat with coconut oil.

7. Carefully release *Gyro Meat* from loaf pan and peel away parchment or aluminum. Use tongs and sharp knife to cut lengthwise into 1/4 inch thick slices.

8. Add sliced meat to hot oiled skillet in single layer and sear about 2 minutes on each side, until browned and lightly crisp. Flip halfway through cooking.

9. Peel and slice red onion. Seed and chop tomato. Transfer romaine lettuce to serving dishes. Layer *Gyro Meat* over lettuce, then top with *Coconut Cream Tzatziki*, onions and tomatoes.

10. Use lettuce to wrap up meat and veggies and serve immediately.

Greek Souvlaki Kebobs

Prep Time: 5 minutes*

Cook Time: 15 minutes

Servings: 4

INGREDIENTS

12 oz (3/4 lb) boneless skinless chicken

1 lemon

2 garlic cloves

1/2 small white onion

1/2 yellow bell pepper

1/2 cup grape tomato

1 teaspoon dried oregano

3/4 teaspoon Celtic sea salt

2 tablespoons coconut oil

8 skewers

INSTRUCTIONS

1. *Soak wooden skewers in water for 10 minutes, if using.
2. Juice lemon into medium mixing bowl. Peel and mince garlic. Remove stem, seeds and veins from bell pepper. Peel onion. Roughly chop pepper and onion. Add to bowl with tomatoes, 1 tablespoon coconut oil, oregano and salt.
3. *Pierce chicken multiple times with fork, then cut into one inch chunks. Add to bowl and mix to combine. Let set aside in refrigerator for 10 minutes.

4. Heat small skillet or griddle over medium-high heat and add 1 tablespoon coconut oil.
5. Drain marinated chicken and veggies, then carefully add to skewer, alternating meat and veggies.
6. Add chicken and veggie skewer to hot oiled skillet or griddle. Grill for about 1 - 2 minutes then turn 1/4 the way around. Continue cooking and turning until chicken is golden brown and cooked through.
7. Remove from heat and serve immediately.

Beef Stuffed Cabbage in Tomato Sauce

Prep Time: 15 minutes

Cook Time: 60 minutes

Servings: 6

INGREDIENTS

1 large cabbage head

Filling

2 1/2 lbs ground beef

4 cage-free eggs

1/2 onion (yellow or white)

1/3 cup almond flour

1/2 cup cauliflower (riced or minced)

1/2 teaspoon dried thyme

1/2 teaspoon ground black pepper (or ground white pepper)

1 1/2 teaspoons Celtic sea salt

Tomato Sauce

2 cans (15 oz) organic tomato sauce

1/2 cup golden raisins

1/2 onion (yellow or white)

2 tablespoons raw honey (or agave or date butter)

2 tablespoons apple cider vinegar

1 1/2 teaspoons Celtic sea salt

1 teaspoon ground black pepper (or ground white pepper)

2 tablespoons bacon fat (or coconut oil or ghee)

INSTRUCTIONS

1. Preheat oven to 350 degrees F. Bring large pot of salted water to boil.

2. Carefully place cabbage head in boiling water for about 5 minutes. Use tongs to peel each layer of leaves from head as soon as they become tender. Set leaves aside on sheet pan to cool.

3. For *Tomato Sauce*, peel and mince onions. Add 1/2 of onions to medium mixing bowl. Add tomato sauce, honey, vinegar, raisins, salt and spices and mix to combine.

4. For *Filling*, add remaining onions to large mixing bowl. Mince or rice cauliflower and add to bowl with eggs, almond flour, salt, spices, and 1 cup *Tomato Sauce*. Mix well with hands or large wooden spoon.

5. Cut hard rib from bottom of each cooled cabbage leaf. Place 1/3 - 1/2 cup *Filling* near the bottom edge of cabbage leaf and roll into a neat package, tucking in sides as you roll. Repeat with remaining filling and cabbage.

6. Spread 1 cup *Tomato sauce* along bottom of deep, lidded baking dish. Place 1/2 the cabbage rolls in baking dish. Add 1/2 remaining sauce, the remaining cabbage rolls. Top with remaining sauce.

7. Tightly cover dish with lid and bake for 1 hour, until meat is cooked through and veggies are tender.

8. Transfer to serving dish and serve hot.

Homestyle Sunday Meatloaf

Prep Time: 10 minutes

Cook Time: 1 hour

Servings: 8

INGREDIENTS

Meatloaf

32 oz (2 lb) ground meat (beef, pork, turkey, chicken, or any combination)

3/4 cup almond flour

2 cage-free eggs

1 medium onion (white, yellow or red)

2 garlic cloves

2 tablespoons oregano

2 tablespoons paprika

1 tablespoon dried thyme

1 tablespoon ground bay leaf (optional)

1 tablespoon ground black pepper

Ketchup

6 oz (1 can) organic tomato paste

3/4 cup water

1 tablespoon apple cider vinegar

1/4 teaspoon garlic powder

1/4 teaspoon onion powder

Pinch all spice (optional)

INSTRUCTIONS

1. Preheat oven to 350 degrees F. Heat small pot over medium heat.

2. For *Ketchup*, add tomato paste, water, apple cider vinegar, garlic powder, onion powder and all spice (optional) to small pot. Reduced for about 5 minutes, stirring occasionally. Remove from heat and set aside.

3. For *Meatloaf*, peel and mince garlic and onion. Or add to food processor and coarsely grind. Add to large mixing bowl.

4. Add eggs to mixing bowl and mix lightly. Add ground meat, almond flour, spices and salt. Mix with hands or large wooden spoon until well combined.

5. Spread a few spoonfuls of *Ketchup* into bottom of medium loaf pan. Transfer meat mixture to loaf pan. Pack slightly and smooth top. Spread 1/2 of *Ketchup* over top of Meatloaf. Cover with aluminum foil and bake for 30 minutes.

6. Carefully remove *Meatloaf* from oven and remove foil. Spread remaining ketchup over *Meatloaf* and continue to bake uncovered for 15 - 30 minutes, until meatloaf is cooked through and Ketchup is caramelized.

7. Remove from oven and let Meatloaf rest about 5 - 10 minutes.

8. Use large spatulas to remove whole *Meatloaf* from pan. Or leave *Meatloaf* in pan, and slice and serve warm.

Brazilian Churrasco with Chimichurri

Prep Time: 10 minutes*

Cook Time: 5 minutes

Servings: 4

INGREDIENTS

24 oz (1 1/2 lb) beef tenderloin

Chimichurri

1 cup coconut oil

1/3 cup apple cider vinegar (or coconut aminos)

1/3 cup water

1 large bunch cilantro

1 large bunch parsley

1/2 cup fresh mint leaves

6 garlic cloves

1/2 teaspoon red pepper flakes

1/2 teaspoon black pepper

1 teaspoon Celtic sea salt

INSTRUCTIONS

1. For *Chimichurri*, peel garlic and add to food processor or high-speed blender. Remove cilantro, parsley and mint leaves from stems. Add to processor and process to finely chop, about 1 minute. Add oil, water, salt and spices. Process until thick sauce forms, about 1 - 2 minutes.

2. Cut tenderloin lengthwise into 4 even slices, then flatten with tenderizing or kitchen mallet to 1/2 inch thickness. Place meat in between two parchment sheets to flatten, if preferred.

3. *Pour 1/4 of the *Chimichurri* into a baking dish just large enough to fit tenderloin. Place beef over *Chimichurri*, then top with second 1/4 of *Chimichurri*. Set aside to marinate about 1 hour. Transfer remaining *Chimichurri* to serving dish.

4. Heat grill or grated skillet over high heat.

5. Place beef on grill or skillet on the diagonal and cook for about 1 minute, then rotate meat to create crosshatch grill marks and cook for another minute. Then flip and repeat. Cook for about 4 minutes total for medium rare.

6. Remove from grill, slice against the grain and transfer to serving dish. Serve immediately with *Chimichurri*.

Holiday Cookbook

Sweet and Tart Cranberry Sauce

Prep Time: 5 minutes

Cook Time: 15 minutes

Servings: 8

INGREDIENTS

24 oz (2 bags) cranberries (fresh or frozen)

1 cup raw honey (or agave or date butter)

2 cups orange juice (about 8 oranges)

INSTRUCTIONS

1.   Heat medium pot over medium-high heat.

2.   Juice oranges and add to pot with sweetener. Stir to combine. Add cranberries and simmer until cranberries start to burst, about 15 minutes.

3.   Remove from heat and transfer to serving dish. Let cool to room temperature, about 30 minutes. Or chill in refrigerator, about 30 minutes.

4.   Serve room temperature or chilled.

"Green Bean" Casserole

Prep Time: 5 minutes

Cook Time: 20 minutes

Servings: 12

INGREDIENTS

Casserole

4 cups asparagus

2 cups button mushrooms

1 cup nut milk

1/2 cup chicken stock

2 tablespoons tapioca flour

1 teaspoon ground white pepper (or ground black pepper)

1 teaspoon garlic powder

1 teaspoon onion powder

Crispy Onions

1/2 cup almond meal

1/2 medium onion (yellow or white)

1 cage-free egg

1 teaspoon paprika

1 teaspoon onion powder

1/4 teaspoon ground black pepper

1 teaspoon Celtic sea salt

Coconut oil (for cooking)

INSTRUCTIONS

1. Preheat oven to 350 degrees F. Bring medium pot of water plus 1/2 teaspoon salt to a boil.

2. For *Casserole*, cut asparagus stalks into quarters. Add to boiling water for about 3 - 4 minutes, until tender but not mushy. Drain and shock in ice bath to stop cooking an preserve color. Set aside.

3. Add tapioca flour and chicken stock to large pan and heat over medium-high heat. Whisk until smooth, then add nut milk, white pepper, garlic and onion powder.

4. Slice mushrooms and add to pan. Stir and thicken about 8 minutes, until thick and creamy.

5. Add asparagus to pan and stir to coat. Pour into baking or casserole dish and bake about 20 minutes, until heated through. Remove from oven and let cool BOUT 5 minutes.

6. Heat medium pan on medium-high heat and coat with coconut oil.

7. For *Crispy Onions*, whisk egg in medium bowl. In shallow dish, mix almond meal with spices.

8. Peel and slice onion. Toss onions in beaten egg, then in seasoned almond meal to coat. Add to hot oiled pan and fry until crispy and golden brown, about 1 - 2 minutes.

9. Drain *Crispy Onions* on paper towel, then sprinkle over *Casserole*. Serve warm.

Tender Collard Greens

Prep Time: 15 minutes

Cook Time: 2 1/2 hours

Servings: 8

INGREDIENTS

2 heads (or 2 large bags) fresh collard greens

6 slices nitrate-free bacon (or 1 small ham hock)

8 cups chicken stock

Water

INSTRUCTIONS

1. Preheat oven to 350 degrees F. Heat large pot over medium-high heat.
2. Rinse collards well and roughly chop. Place in large colander or in clean sink to drain.
3. Add bacon or ham hock to hot pot and render down for about 5 minutes.
4. Add greens to pot in batches. If all greens to not fit, reserve. Add chicken stock.
5. Bring pot to a simmer then reduce to low heat. Add any remaining greens, plus enough water just to cover, if necessary. Stir gently.
6. Simmer until collards are tender, about 2 - 2 1/2 hours.
7. Drain greens well. Transfer to serving dish and serve warm.

Christmas Skillet "Cornbread"

Prep Time: 5 minutes

Cook Time: 25 minutes

Servings: 12

INGREDIENTS

1 2/3 cups almond flour

3 cage-free eggs

1/3 cup coconut oil (or coconut or cacao butter, melted)

1/3 cup nut milk

2 tablespoons organic apple cider vinegar

2 teaspoons baking powder

1/2 teaspoon ground turmeric or mustard (optional)

1/2 teaspoon ground white pepper (or ground black pepper)

Coconut oil (for cooking)

INSTRUCTIONS

1. Preheat oven to 350 degrees F. Lightly coat cast-iron pan or skillet with coconut oil. Place in oven to heat pan.

2. Beat eggs in medium mixing bowl with hand mixer or whisk until thick and slightly frothy, about 1 minute. Add oil or butter, nut milk and vinegar. Mix well.

3. Beat in almond meal, baking powder and spices until combined. Batter should be thick and moist. Add nut milk to thin, if necessary.

4. Remove pan from oven. Carefully pour batter into hot oiled pan and bake 25 - 30 minutes, until edges are golden brown and top is firm. Remove from oven.

5. Slice and serve warm. Or allow to cool completely and serve room temperature.

Sage "Cornbread" Dressing

Prep Time: 10 minutes*

Cook Time: 30 minutes

Servings: 12

INGREDIENTS

Skillet Cornbread

Roasted Turkey (optional)

8 oz all-natural sausage (spicy or sweet)

2 celery stalks

2 teaspoons ground sage

1 - 2 cups chicken stock

INSTRUCTIONS

1. *Chop *Skillet Cornbread* and let dry in open air, overnight to 24 hours.

2. Preheat oven to 350 degrees F. Lightly coat baking dish or with coconut oil. Heat medium pan or skillet over medium heat.

3. Remove sausage from casing, crumble and add to hot pan. Dice celery and add to sausage. Sauté until sausage is browned and celery is a bit tender, about 5 - 8 minutes.

4. Add chicken stock to hot pan and stir with wooden spoon to deglaze pam. Remove from heat.

5. Add chopped dried *Skillet Cornbread* to large mixing bowl. Use slotted spoon to scoop sausage and celery into bowl. Pour about half of chicken stock over cornbread mixture.

6. Add ground sage and mix with hand or large wooden spoon. Mix until cornbread is fully moistened but not soggy. Add chicken stock as necessary.

7. Transfer mixture to baking dish or pan and bake 30 - 35 minutes, until golden brown and firm, but still moist.

8. Or stuff *Roasted Turkey* and cook about 18 - 20 minutes per lb.

9. Remove from oven and serve warm.

Sweet Candied Yams

Prep Time: 10 minutes

Cook Time: 1 hour 30 minutes

Servings: 12

INGREDIENTS

4 large sweet potatoes (yams)

1/2 cup dried pitted dates

1/4 cup dried apricots

2 tablespoons coconut butter (or cacao butter or ghee)

1 tablespoon ground cinnamon

1/2 teaspoon ground ginger

1/2 teaspoon ground black pepper (or ground white pepper) (optional)

Pinch Celtic sea salt

Topping

1/2 cup pecan pieces (or 1 cup pecan halves)

1/4 cup raw honey (or agave or date butter)

INSTRUCTIONS

1. Preheat oven to 350 degrees F.
2. Gently rinse sweet potatoes and place on sheet pan.
3. Bake about 1 hour, until tender.
4. Add dates, apricots and enough water to cover in small pot. Heat over medium heat. Let simmer until water evaporates. Remove from heat.
5. Remove yams from oven and let cool about 10 minutes.

6. For *Topping*, add pecans and sweetener to small pan. Heat over medium heat and cook until pecans are lightly toasted and caramelized, about 4 - 5 minutes. Stir frequently and do not burn. Remove from heat and set aside.

7. Add softened dates and apricots to large mixing bowl. Mash with potato masher, hand mixer or whisk.

8. Cut yams open lengthwise and scoop flesh into mixing bowl. Add butter, salt and spices. Mash with potato masher, hand mixer or whisk until well combined.

9. Transfer yam mixture to serving dish and top with *Topping*. Serve warm.

Pineapple Spice Baked Ham

Prep Time: 10 minutes

Cook Time: 5 hours

Servings: 12

INGREDIENTS

1 (12 lb) bone-in ham

1 (20 oz) can organic pineapple rings (in juice)

1/2 cup date butter (or raw honey or agave)

1/2 cup whole cloves

1/2 cup water

1 lemon

1 lime

1 orange

About 12 pitted cherries (optional)

Toothpicks (optional)

INSTRUCTIONS

1. Preheat oven to 325 degrees F.

2. Drain pineapple juice into small mixing bowl. Juice lemon, lime and orange into bowl. Add sweetener and water. Mix well.

3. Place ham in roasting pan and score rind in crosshatch (diamond) pattern with knife.

4. Press cloves into rind. Place cherries on rind and secure with toothpick. Hang pineapple rings on cherries.

5. Pour pineapple juice mixture over ham and bake uncovered 4 - 5 hours, until internal temperature reaches 160 degrees F. Baste with juices about every 30 minutes.

6. Remove ham from oven. Remove toothpicks and carve. Serve hot.

Perfect Roasted Turkey

Prep Time: 10 minutes*

Cook Time: 4 - 6 hours

Servings: 12

INGREDIENTS

20 lb (approx.) whole turkey

1 teaspoon paprika (or smoked paprika or Hungarian paprika)

2 teaspoons Celtic sea salt

2 teaspoons ground black pepper

2 tablespoons coconut oil

Brine

1 - 2 gallons water

1 cup Celtic sea salt

1 cup raw honey (or agave or date butter)

INSTRUCTIONS

1. *For *Brine*, add 1/2 gallon of water, salt and sweetener to large baking dish or roasting pan. Mix to combine. Remove any entrails from turkey and add to *Brine*, plus and enough water to submerge completely. Marinate in refrigerator 12 - 24 hours.

2. Preheat oven to 350 degrees F. Place roasting rack in clean roasting pan.

3. Drain turkey and rub salt, pepper, paprika and oil over and under skin, where possible.

4. Place seasoned turkey on roasting rack and bake about 15 - 18 minutes per lb, about 5 hours for 20 lb bird. Or until internal temperature reaches 165 degrees F. Baste with rendered fat and juices throughout cooking for even browning.
5. Remove turkey from oven and let rest 20 - 30 minutes.
6. Carve and serve warm.

Homestyle Sweet Potato Pie

Prep Time: 10 minutes

Cook Time: 50 minutes

Servings: 6

INGREDIENTS

Crust

2 cups almond flour

1 cage-free egg

2 tablespoons coconut oil (or cacao butter or ghee)

1/4 teaspoon Celtic sea salt

Filling

2 cups organic canned yams (mashed)

2 cage-free eggs

1/2 cup date butter (or raw honey or agave)

1/2 cup coconut oil (or coconut or cacao butter)

1/2 cup nut milk

2 teaspoons cinnamon

1 teaspoon vanilla

1/4 teaspoon nutmeg

Water

INSTRUCTIONS

1. Preheat oven to 350 degrees F.

2. For *Crust*, blend almond flour and salt in small mixing bowl. Add egg and oil or butter. Mix until dough forms. Press into pie pan with hand or wooden spoon. Set aside.

3. For *Filling*, add mashed yams, eggs, oil or butter, sweetener, cinnamon, nutmeg and vanilla to food processor or high-speed blender with nut milk. Process until smooth, about 1 minute. Process until smooth, about 1 - 2 minutes.

4. Pour batter into *Crust* and bake about 45 - 50 minutes, or until center is set.

5. Remove from oven and let cool about 20 minutes.

6. Slice and serve warm. Or let cool completely and serve room temperature.

Holiday Apple Crumble

Prep Time: 20 minutes

Cook Time: 50 minutes

Servings: 8

INGREDIENTS

Crust

2 cups almond flour

1 cage-free egg

2 tablespoons coconut oil (or cacao butter or ghee)

1/4 teaspoon Celtic sea salt

Filling

5 apples

1/2 cup date butter (or raw honey or agave)

1/2 lemon

1 teaspoon ground cinnamon

1/2 teaspoon vanilla

1/4 teaspoon ground nutmeg

1/4 teaspoon Celtic sea salt

Topping

1/2 cup almond flour

1/2 cup pecans

1/2 cup shredded coconut

1/4 cup cold cacao butter (or coconut butter, ghee or coconut oil)

1/4 cup raw honey (or agave)

1/4 cup dried pitted dates

2 tablespoons ground flax

1 teaspoon cinnamon

INSTRUCTIONS

1. Preheat oven to 375 degrees F.
2. For *Crust*, blend almond flour and salt in small mixing bowl. Add egg and oil or butter. Mix until dough forms. Press into pie pan or baking dish with hand or wooden spoon. Set aside.
3. For *Filling*, core and peel apples. Cut into thin slices and add to large mixing bowl. Add sweetener, salt and spices. Juice 1/2 lemon over apples and mix to combine. Press apples firmly into *Crust*.
4. For *Topping*, add dates and honey or agave to food processor or high-speed blender. Process until coarsely ground, about 1 minute. Add butter or oil, almond flour, pecans, coconut, flax and cinnamon. Pulse until finely chopped or coarsely ground. Sprinkle *Topping* over apples.
5. Bake 40 - 50 minutes, until apples are cooked and *Topping* is browned and crisp.
6. Remove from oven and allow to cool at least 5 minutes.
7. Slice and serve warm. Or let cool completed and serve room temperature.

Delicious Fruit Cake

Prep Time: 10 minutes

Cook Time: 40 minutes

Servings: 8

INGREDIENTS

1 1/2 cups almond flour

4 cage-free eggs

1/2 cup chopped walnuts (or 3/4 walnuts halves)

1 orange

1/4 cup raw honey (or agave or date butter)

2 tablespoons coconut oil (coconut or cacao butter, melted)

1/2 cup dried pitted dates

1/2 cup dried cherries

1/2 cup dried apricots

1/2 cup raisins

1/2 teaspoon baking soda

1 teaspoon ground ginger

1 teaspoon vanilla

1/2 teaspoon Celtic sea salt

INSTRUCTIONS

1. Preheat oven to 350 degrees F. Lightly medium loaf pan or round cake pan with coconut oil, or line with parchment paper.

2. Sift almond flour, baking soda and salt into large mixing bowl. Chop apricots, dates and walnut halves , if using. Add to flour mixture with dried cherries and raisins.

3. Zest *then* juice orange into medium mixing bowl. Add eggs, oil or butter, sweetener, ginger and vanilla. Beat with hand mixer or whisk until well combined.
4. Pour egg mixture into flour mixture. Mix to combine.
5. Transfer batter to prepared loaf or cake pan and smooth top with spatula.
6. Bake 35 - 40 minutes, until browned and toothpick inserted into center comes out clean.
7. Remove from oven and allow to cool at least 10 minutes.
8. Slice and serve warm. Or let cool completely and serve room temperature.

Sweet Pumpkin Cheesecake

Prep Time: 15 minutes*

Cook Time: 10 Minutes

Servings: 12

INGREDIENTS

Crust

1/2 cup coconut flour

1/4 cup cacao butter (or coconut butter or coconut oil)

1/4 cup raw honey (or agave or date butter)

1/2 cup shredded or flaked coconut

Filling

1 1/2 cups raw cashews

1 cup organic pumpkin purée

1/2 cup date butter (or agave or raw honey)

1/2 cup full-fat coconut milk

1/2 cup coconut oil (or cacao or coconut butter, melted)

1 lemon

1 1/2 teaspoons vanilla

2 teaspoons ground cinnamon

1/2 teaspoon ground nutmeg

1/4 teaspoon ground clove

1/4 teaspoon ground ginger

1/2 teaspoon Celtic sea salt

Water

INSTRUCTIONS

1. *For *Filling*, soak cashews in enough water to cover for at least 4 hours to overnight in refrigerator. Drain and rinse.

2. Preheat oven to 375 degrees F.

3. For *Crust*, place all ingredients in food processor or high-speed blender. Process until well ground and mixture sticks together, about 2 minutes.

4. Press *Crust* firmly into bottom of spring form pan with hands. Bake about 8 minutes, then set aside.

5. For *Filling*, zest *then* juice lemon into clean food processor or high-speed blender. Add soaked cashews, pumpkin purée, sweetener, coconut milk, oil or butter, vanilla, salt and spices. Process until smooth, about 2 - 3 minutes.

6. Pour *Filling* into *Crust* and smooth with spatula.

7. *Cover pie with parchment, if preferred, and set aside in refrigerator at least 4 hours to set.

8. Slice and serve chilled.

Harvest Spice Cake

Prep Time: 10 minutes

Cook Time: 40 minutes

Servings: 8

INGREDIENTS

1 cup almond flour

1/2 cup coconut flour

3 cage-free eggs (separated)

1/4 cup coconut oil (or coconut or cacao butter, melted)

1/4 - 1/3 cup raw honey (or agave or date butter)

1/4 cup unsweetened applesauce

1/4 cup nut milk

1 orange

1 teaspoon baking soda

1 tablespoon ground cinnamon

1 tablespoon ground ginger

1 teaspoon ground nutmeg

1 teaspoon vanilla

1 teaspoon ground black pepper

1/2 teaspoon Celtic sea salt

INSTRUCTIONS

1. Preheat oven to 350 degrees F. Coat round cake pan, square baking dish or medium loaf pan with coconut oil, or line with parchment paper.

2. Sift almond and coconut flour, baking soda, salt and spices into large mixing bowl.

3. In medium mixing bowl, beat egg whites to soft peaks with hand mixer or whisk, about 5 minutes.

4. Zest *then* juice orange into egg whites. Beat in egg yolks, oil or butter, nut milk, sweetener and applesauce. Add egg mixture to flour mixture and mix until combined.

5. Pour batter into prepared pan and bake for 35 - 40 minutes, until browned and firm but springy in the center. Toothpick inserted into center should come out clean.

6. Remove from oven and allow to cool at least 5 - 10 minutes.

7. Slice and serve warm. Or let cool completely and serve room temperature.

Sweet Date Gingerbread Cookies

Prep Time: 5 minutes

Cook Time: 15 minutes

Servings: 12

INGREDIENTS

1 cup almond flour

2 cage-free eggs

1/2 cup dried pitted dates

1/4 cup raw honey (or dark agave)

1/4 cup coconut oil (or cacao butter, melted)

1/2 teaspoon baking soda

1/2 teaspoon baking powder

2 teaspoons ground ginger

1 teaspoon ground cinnamon

1 teaspoon vanilla

1/2 teaspoon ground cloves

1/2 teaspoon ground black pepper

1/4 teaspoon Celtic sea salt

Natural sarsaparilla or root beer beverage, or nut milk (optional)

INSTRUCTIONS

1. Preheat oven to 350 degrees F. Line sheet pan with parchment or baking mat.

2. Add dates, honey or agave and eggs to food processor or high-speed blender. Process until thick smooth mixture forms, about 2 minutes.

3. Add almond flour, oil or butter, baking soda and powder, salt and spices to processor. Process until thick mixture comes together, about 1 minute. Add sarsaparilla, root beer or nut milk to thin as necessary. Batter should resemble thick cookie dough.

4. From rounds and place on prepares sheet pan. Flatten into disks.

5. Bake 10 - 15 minutes, until browned around edges and cooked through, but still soft.

6. Remove from oven and let cool at about 10 minutes.

7. Transfer to serving dish and serve warm. Or cool completely and serve room temperature.

Warm Spiced Mulled Wine

Prep Time: 5 minutes

Cook Time: 15 minutes

Servings: 4

INGREDIENTS

4 cups apple cider

1 (750 ml) bottle red wine

1/4 cup raw honey (or agave or stevia)

1 orange

2 whole cinnamon sticks

4 whole cloves

3 whole star anise pods

INSTRUCTIONS

1. Zest then juice orange into medium-large pot. Add wine, apple cider, sweetener and whole spices.
2. Bring to a boil, then reduce heat to low. Simmer 10 minutes.
3. Pour into serving glasses and serve warm.

Coconut Milk Eggnog

Prep Time: 5 minutes*

Cook Time: 15 minutes

Servings: 4

INGREDIENTS

4 cage-free egg yolks

2 (14 oz) cans organic full-fat coconut milk

1/3 cup raw honey (or agave or date butter)

1/2 teaspoon ground nutmeg

1/2 teaspoon ground cinnamon

Nut milk (optional)

Rum, to taste (optional)

INSTRUCTIONS

1. Add coconut milk to medium pot and heat over medium heat. Bring to simmer, stirring occasionally.

2. Add egg yolks to medium mixing bowl. Beat with hand mixer or whisk until light and frothy, about 5 minutes. Beat in sweetener.

3. Slowly beat a few tablespoons hot coconut milk into eggs to temper. Do not scramble. Slowly add remaining coconut milk and beat well to combine.

4. Pour mixture back into hot pot. Add spices and simmer until thickened, about 5 - 8 minutes. Stir frequently.

5. *Remove from heat and stir in rum (optional). Transfer to glass container and chill in refrigerator at least 1 hour.

6. Add nut milk to thin to desired consistency (optional). Pour into serving glasses and serve chilled.

Sweet Horchata

Prep Time: 5 minutes*

Servings: 4

INGREDIENTS

5 cups water

1 1/2 cups shredded or flaked coconut

1/2 cup full-fat coconut milk

1/2 cup raw honey (or agave or stevia)

2 teaspoons vanilla

2 teaspoons ground cinnamon

INSTRUCTIONS

1. *Add shredded coconut and water high-speed blender and process about 1 minute. Transfer mixture to container and set aside in refrigerator 2 - 4 hours.

2. Strain mixture into serving container. Add full-fat coconut milk, sweetener, vanilla and cinnamon. Stir to combine.

3. Serve chilled.

Sweet Mango Lassi

Prep Time: 5 minutes

Servings: 2

INGREDIENTS

2 ripe mangos

2 cups full-fat coconut milk (or kefir)

1 cup ice

1/4 - 1/2 cup raw honey (or agave, date butter or stevia) (optional)

INSTRUCTIONS

1. Add ice and coconut milk to high-speed blender. Pulse to crush ice.
2. Cut mango around pit. Remove peel and cut into chunks. Add to blender with sweetener (optional). Process until smooth, about 1 minute.
3. Pour into glasses and serve immediately.

Pan Asian Mushroom Masala

Prep Time: 10 minutes

Cook Time: 25 minutes

Servings: 8

INGREDIENTS

1 head cauliflower

1 1/2 cups tomato purée (or tomato sauce)

1 pint (2 cups) mushrooms

1 onion

1 chili pepper

1 /2 green bell pepper

1 large garlic clove

1 inch piece fresh ginger

2 teaspoons coriander leaves (optional)

1 teaspoon garam masala

1/2 teaspoon cayenne pepper

1/2 teaspoon ground coriander

1/2 teaspoon Celtic sea salt

3 tablespoons bacon fat (or coconut oil or ghee)

INSTRUCTIONS

1. Roughly chop cauliflower, then rice cauliflower in food processor, or mince. Add to medium pot with enough water to cover. Heat pot over medium heat and cook until just tender, about 8 minutes. Drain and transfer to serving dish.

2. Heat medium pan over medium heat. Add bacon fat, oil or butter to hot pan.
3. Peel and finely dice onions. Remove seeds, veins and stem from bell pepper and dice. Slice chili pepper. Peel and mince garlic and onion. Add to hot oiled pan and sauté about 5 minutes.
4. Slice mushrooms and add to pan with tomato, salt and spices. Finely chop coriander leaves and add to pan (optional). Sauté and let simmer about 10 - 12 minutes, stirring occasionally.
5. Transfer to serving dish and serve hot with cauliflower rice.

Indian Sweet Fig Pudding

Prep Time: 10 minutes*

Cook Time: 4 Hours

Servings: 8

INGREDIENTS

3 cage-free eggs

1 1/2 cups figs (fresh or dried)

1/2 cup shredded or flaked coconut

1/3 cup coconut flour

1/3 cup date butter (or agave or raw honey)

1 cup coconut milk

1/2 teaspoon ground nutmeg

Coconut oil (or cacao butter or ghee)

INSTRUCTIONS

1. Soak dried dates in enough water to cover for at least 2 hours, if using. Drain.

2. Preheat oven to 350 degrees F. Coat baking dish well with oil or butter.

3. Beat eggs and coconut milk in medium mixing bowl. Add coconut flour, shredded coconut, sweetener and nutmeg. Mix well.

4. Chop figs and add to bowl. Mix to combine.

5. Transfer mixture to prepared baking dish and smooth top with spatula or knife.

6. Set baking dish in larger dish or roasting pan and place in oven. Fill larger vessel with water 3/4 of the way up baking dish.

7. Tightly cover larger vessel with lid or aluminum foil and bake 3 - 4 hours, until *Fig Pudding* is set and cooked through.

8. Carefully remove baking dish from larger vessel, and from oven. Let cool at least 10 minutes.

9. Slice and serve warm.

Asian Holiday Spiced Nuts

Prep Time: 5 minutes

Cook Time: 25 minutes

Servings: 8

INGREDIENTS

1 cup raw almonds

1/2 cup raw walnuts

1/2 cup raw cashews

1/2 cup raw pistachios

2 - 4 tablespoons raw honey (or agave or date butter)

1 teaspoon paprika (or smoked paprika or Hungarian paprika)

1/2 teaspoon ground cumin

1/2 teaspoon ground black pepper

1/2 teaspoon Chinese 5-spice blend (optional)

1/2 teaspoon all spice (optional)

1 teaspoon Celtic sea salt

2 tablespoons ghee (or bacon fat, cocoa butter or coconut oil)

INSTRUCTIONS

1. Heat cast iron pan or skillet over medium-high heat. Add ghee, butter or oil to hot pan.

2. Add nuts to hot oiled pan and. Stir continuously and sauté until lightly browned and aromatic, about 2 - 3 minutes.

3. Add salt, spices and sweetener to pan and sauté until caramelized, about 5 minutes. Stir continuously and do not burn.

4. Transfer nuts to sheet pan and spread in single layer to cool at least 5 minutes.
5. Transfer to serving dish and serve warm. Or cool completely and serve room temperature.

French Holiday Tapenade

Prep Time: 15 minutes

Servings: 2

INGREDIENTS

1 1/2 cups any combination pitted olives (Kalamata, Spanish, black, pimento, etc.)

2 tablespoons capers

2 anchovy fillets

1 garlic clove

2 fresh basil leaves

1/2 lemon

2 tablespoons coconut oil

INSTRUCTIONS

1. Peel garlic and add to food processor or high-speed blender. Process until finely ground.
2. Rinse and drain olives, capers and anchovy fillets. Add to processor with basil, oil and squeeze of 1/2 lemon. Process until finely chopped or coarsely ground, about 1 - 2 minutes.
3. Transfer to serving dish and serve immediately.

Hanukkah Sweet Potato Latkes

Prep Time: 10 minutes

Cook Time: 20 minutes

Servings: 4

INGREDIENTS

1 large sweet potato

1/2 onion (yellow or white)

2 cage-free eggs

1/2 teaspoon ground black pepper

1/2 teaspoon Celtic sea salt

 1 cup organic unsweetened applesauce (optional)

Coconut oil (for cooking)

Water

INSTRUCTIONS

1. Heat large pan or skillet over medium heat. Lightly coat hot pan with oil.

2. Peel sweet potato and onion, then grate with grater or shredding attachment in food processor.

3. Line medium mixing bowl with paper towels. Add onions and squeeze out as much water as possible. Remove paper towels.

4. Add sweet potatoes to separate mixing bowl. Add enough water to cover potatoes plus salt. Mix then rinse starch from potatoes. Drain in colander, then on paper towels.

5. Add rinsed sweet potatoes to onions with eggs and pepper. Mix to combine.

6. Add sweet potato mixture to hot oiled pan in heaping tablespoons. Flatten patties with fork. Brown 5 - 8 minutes on one side, then flip with spatula. Cook another 5 - 8 minutes until cooked through and crisp. Drain on paper towels.

7. Transfer to serving dish and serve hot with applesauce (optional).

Lots o' Matzo Ball Soup

Prep Time: 5 minutes*

Cook Time: 10 minutes

Servings: 6

INGREDIENTS

6 cups chicken stock (or vegetable stock)

2 cups almond flour

4 cage-free egg yolks

1/4 teaspoon ground white pepper (or ground black pepper)

2 teaspoons Celtic sea salt

INSTRUCTIONS

1. In a medium bowl, beat eggs,1 teaspoon salt and pepper until light and frothy, about 2 minutes. Sift almond flour into bowl and mix until dough comes together.

2. *Cover dough with parchment, if preferred, and refrigerate 2 - 4 hours.

3. Add 1 teaspoon salt to large pot of water and bring to boil. Add chicken stock to medium pot and heat over medium heat.

4. Remove dough from refrigerator and roll into balls. Carefully place dough balls in boiling water. Reduce heat to low, cover and simmer 20 minutes, until cooked through.

5. Transfer matzo balls to serving dish with slotted spoon. Ladle heated chicken stock over matzo balls and serve hot.

Festival Cherry Nut Rugelach

Prep Time: 25 minutes

Cook Time: 25 minutes

Servings: 12

INSTRUCTIONS

Crust

2 cups almond flour

2 cage-free eggs

2 tablespoons coconut oil

2 tablespoons cacao butter, melted (or full-fat coconut milk)

2 tablespoons raw honey (or agave or date butter)

1 teaspoon baking powder

1/2 teaspoon baking soda

1/2 teaspoon vanilla

1/4 teaspoon ground cinnamon

1/4 teaspoon ground ginger

1/4 teaspoon Celtic sea salt

Filling

1/2 cup dried cherries

1/2 cup walnuts

1/2 cup raw honey (or agave or date butter)

2 tablespoons ghee, melted (or cacao or coconut butter, melted)

1/2 teaspoon cinnamon

1/2 teaspoon ginger

Pinch Celtic sea salt

Splash of Brandy (optional)

INSTRUCTIONS

1. For *Crust*, sift almond flour into medium mixing bowl. Add baking soda and powder, vanilla, cinnamon, ginger and salt.
2. Whisk eggs and sweetener in small mixing bowl, then add to flour mixture and combine. Slowly add coconut oil and cacao butter or coconut milk until malleable dough comes together.
3. Roll in plastic wrap or wrap tightly in parchment and refrigerate for 15 minutes.
4. Preheat oven to 325 degrees F. Line sheet pan with parchment or baking mat. Cover cutting board with parchment. Heat medium pan over medium heat.
5. For *Filling*, add walnuts to dry hot pan and toast about 2 minutes, stirring frequently.
6. Add ghee, sweetener, cherries, salt, spices and splash of Brandy (optional) to walnuts. Stir to combine and heat through, about 1 - 2 minutes. Remove from heat and set aside to cool.
7. Remove dough from refrigerator. Roll dough out on parchment covered cutting board to about 1/4 inch thick rectangle with rolling pin.
8. Spread *Filling* over dough. Use sharp knife or pizza cutter to cut dough into about 12 rectangles.
9. Roll up dough pieces and arrange on prepared sheet pan. Bake 20 - 25 minutes, until dough is golden brown and cooked through.
10. Remove from oven and let cool about 5 minutes.
11. Serve warm. Or allow to cool completely and serve room temperature.